Modeling:
Totally Exposed

Modeling:
Totally Exposed

Marsha Doll-Faulkenberry, Author
Edited by Susan L. Trainor
Cover Design by Gregory Group
Cover Photography by Mark Hanson and
Stephen Leukanech/ Twin Palms Studio

Marsha Doll & Associates
Tallahassee, Florida

To my husband, Dean, my children, Tiffany, Gracie, Sara, and Dean II, my parents and my many friends who have helped me to achieve success. A special thanks to my good friend, Brad Ray, for his guidance and support.

I also wish to express special gratitude to my friends Anna Johnson, Nancy Dignon and Kerey Carpenter as well as so many of my wonderful models.

Additionally, I wish to acknowledge the countless people in my community who have been there for me throughout the development of this book.

TABLE OF CONTENTS

Plus Models
Petite Models
Specialty Models
Male Models

ABOUT THE AUTHOR...
MARSHA DOLL-FAULKENBERRY

Marsha Doll-Faulkenberry, like many other people, grew up dreaming of a glamorous career in the modeling industry. Born in the small, Florida town of Perry, Marsha participated in community fashion shows and other similar events throughout her childhood, always hoping to become a professional model. At

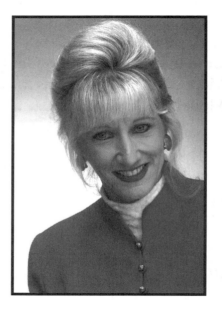

15, she traveled to the Merchandising Mart in Atlanta, Georgia, as a buyer for her parents' clothing store. This experience as a "buyer" led to Marsha's becoming a showroom model at the Mart.

Marsha went to Florida State University to begin her college career in communications. While in Tallahassee, she enrolled in her first modeling school. Marsha excelled in her modeling courses, and she became a part-time instructor of runway, photography and TV commercial courses. She participated as a model in the annual *Models of the South Convention* in Hilton Head Island, South Carolina. Over the years, she has won numerous awards at this convention, and so did the models she instructed. Gradually, Marsha began to understand that her goal was to help prospective models discover their hidden potential.

Marsha received her degree in communications with a minor in psychology from Florida State University. After working with models in Miami and Tampa, Marsha returned to her roots. She opened two modeling agencies — one in her hometown of Perry and one in Tallahassee. She teaches, coaches and promotes models from ages five to 65. Some of her models have been seen in fashion magazines such as *Vogue, Cosmopolitan, Teen, Seventeen,* and *Glamour,* as well as, billboards, film, television commercials and catalogs. She has appeared in films with Brooke Shields, Melanie Griffith, Don Johnson, Eddie Albert, Diana Scarwid, and Jeff Daniels. Marsha Doll educates people interested in the modeling business by way of lectures, seminars and radio and television talk shows. The Marsha Doll Agency has been awarded "Agency of the Year" for five consecutive years.

Today, Marsha lives with her husband, Dean, and their children, in Tallahassee, Florida. Marsha's main purpose in writing this book is to instruct hopeful models in the best, most productive ways to enter the modeling industry. She hopes to influence them to try their hardest to succeed in a very difficult career. In fact, her greatest pleasure is to see the models she has trained and guided become rising stars in an increasingly competitive world.

INTRODUCTION

Welcome to the world of modeling!

The modeling industry is a fast-paced and competitive career choice. It offers excitement and tremendous potential for development, but aspiring models can face serious problems due to their lack of knowledge about modeling. So much beauty goes unnoticed simply because people don't know where to begin. If you decide to become a model, you will face some serious choices. You need to know what to do in each situation.

If you read this book carefully, you may avoid many of the pitfalls that plagued other well-qualified men and women who struggled to get where they are today! I wrote this book to help you use your time and money wisely. It will explain the many different avenues you can take to begin a career in modeling. Also provided is a directory of modeling schools and agencies located throughout the United States. Use this list to target various agencies and schools for interviews, correspondence and personal visits.

I want to educate you because it is imperative that you understand the modeling business and what it takes to succeed. The best way to accomplish this is to combine honesty with my years of real modeling experience. Whether you intend to model professionally or to improve your image and your self-confidence, this book will help you achieve your goals. Your own motivation and drive to succeed are your greatest assets.

Good Luck,

Marsha Doll - Faulkenberry

CAN I REALLY BECOME A MODEL?

Have you ever watched a television commercial and thought, "I <u>know</u> I could do that. I look as good as they do." Or maybe you've seen a print advertisement for a local department store, a fashion show or a magazine advertisement. You know you could do it — but how do you break in? What does it take to be a model? Where do you start?

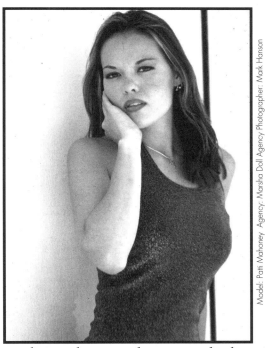

Model: Patti Mahoney Agency: Marsha Doll Agency Photographer: Mark Hanson

My agency receives over 300 phone calls a month from people asking the same questions: "How can I get my baby on a Pampers®commercial?" or "How do models get into catalogs such as J.C. Penney or Sears?" I am very honest with people when answering their questions. The fact is, you have to be where the action is. National TV commercials and catalogs are not being shot anywhere near the location of my agency or in markets of comparable size. Clients located in larger markets rarely call my agency looking for models. You have to live in a big city where these types of clients and agencies exist. When I find someone who I believe has potential to model professionally, I place him or her with another agency in a larger commercial market. That's the only way to get the "big jobs."

It is virtually impossible to make a living modeling in a small town. The only thing you can gain working in a small market is experience and some extra spending money. So please understand, if this sounds like your current situation, you will have to make a change if modeling is to be your career.

The intrigue and glamour of modeling attracts thousands of people who want to know how to get started. It can be an exciting career. Modeling can be a fun and rewarding way of life. But first, you must learn exactly how to deal with the pressures and demands of a career with high visibility. And you must realize that modeling is work! It will never be easy. This book will help you get started. With a lot of effort and some common sense, you, too, can become a model.

Chapter 1
Training & Experience

TRAINING & EXPERIENCE

Modeling Schools

The foundation for a career in modeling may start with assistance from a reputable modeling school. Defining "reputable", however, can be difficult! You should do some extensive research into the backgrounds of prospective schools before making a definite commitment. It is best to look for a school that is affiliated directly with an agency, so when you finish your courses, you'll have that agency connection.

Modeling schools should build your confidence, poise and give you a general understanding of the modeling industry. You must be your own judge when it comes to choosing the school that seems the most professional. Whether you're doing this to feel better about yourself or are truly serious about becoming a professional model, only you will know which courses, instructors and classes will best suit your needs. However, please be certain you have carefully considered the following advice before making your ultimate choice.

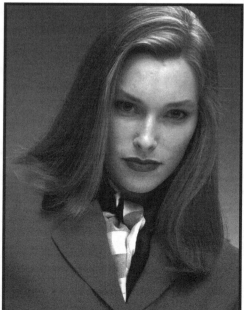

Model: Emily Fletcher Agency: Marsha Doll Agency
Photographer: Stephen Leukanech/ Twin Palms Studio

You do not have to spend a fortune to become a model. Some modeling schools expect you to pay thousands of dollars for their courses. This often involves drawn-out lessons over a long period of time, taking you through what they may refer to as beginning, intermediate, advanced and professional modeling classes. These schools may even require payment of other exorbitant fees for "extras" such as photo shoots. It is important to remember that training and pictures do not have to cost a lot of money and are not necessary. Generally, you should not pay a higher hourly rate for modeling lessons than you would for piano or dance lessons in your area, and it should not take longer than 12 months to complete the course. You can expect to pay a few hundred dollars for modeling school tuition and a modest sum for the tools you need to get started. Be cautious of anyone who suggests that you must pay outrageous fees to reach your goals, and do not sign a school contract that makes you feel uncomfortable. Shop around. Visit different schools. Meet the instructors. Meet the students. Ask if you can take or watch a lesson. Attend a local show where a school's models are working. Here are the key things to look for...

A good modeling school will be interested in you as a person — not only as a prospective student. A modeling school should teach proper etiquette, correct conduct and a sense of personal style, as well as runway, photography and TV commercial courses. Modeling school graduates should have gained confidence and poise upon completion of the course. If a modeling career is your goal, ask the directors of each school for the names of their graduates who have become professionals, as well as, the names of the agencies they work with in the larger markets. This will tell you: 1) how much exposure and attention you can expect to receive; 2) the quality of the school; and 3) whether you will get the experience you need to build your confidence. Of course, just because a school has several famous graduates doesn't mean that you also will become a professional model. But it is nice to follow in the footsteps of success!

A reputable school will give you information pertaining to their national or regional achievements — any school that hesitates to share this information probably isn't worth your time. The Better Business Bureau can be helpful in clearing up any confusion you may have about a particular school's reputation. Also, some states require an agency/school to be licensed. You can call your state agency that regulates business licenses to find out if this is required by law.

Your choice of a school will depend on many different factors. I imagine that the most important consideration is where you currently live. Some of us have fewer choices simply because we live in a smaller town or in a less developed part of the country. Don't let that discourage you! No matter where you live, attending a modeling school does not guarantee that you will become a successful, professional model. (And NOT attending a modeling school does not doom you to failure, either!) A school director would be very unprofessional if he or she told you that your success is "guaranteed".

Your choice either to attend a school or travel straight to markets like New York, Miami or Dallas will have to rest squarely on your own shoulders, because you are the only one who is most aware of your particular situation. One piece of advice, however, there are many modeling schools out there simply trying to "make a buck". Providing you with the best teachers and resources is simply not a priority to them. So, if you choose to attend a school, please be certain that you have made a well-informed, economically sound decision.

A major contribution to the learning process that modeling schools can offer is exposure. You will need to accumulate experience in fashion shows, photo sessions, local television shows, local industrial films and print work in local publications and newspapers. If your school director is a motivated individual, chances are excellent that you will gain familiarity with several different types of modeling assignments. Experience is the "key" to looking and feeling like you are in control in difficult situations, and a good modeling school can provide this assurance for you. But please remember, if anyone promises or guarantees you a modeling job upon completion of their courses — beware. Modeling schools are basically for building confidence, self-esteem and poise and learning beauty and fashion tips. No agency involvement usually means no jobs.

A modeling school needs a motivated, excited director to make things happen for you! Usually, a school with a lazy, uncaring owner suffers from his or her lack of direction — and so do the models, because they don't get the attention they deserve. Look for a school with a director who wants to help you do your best.

Modeling Agencies

My agency is in a small marketplace, but it is large enough to keep me very busy. The population is about 150,000. We provide models for advertising agencies and production companies, as well as, put on fashion shows for local malls. In a market like mine, there is little demand for high-fashion jobs. We hold open calls weekly for people interested in modeling. It's always an adventure to see and meet the types of people who walk through my doors. It amazes the tall, thin, beautiful girls when a 45 to 55 year old, semi-attractive woman walks in, and I literally jump up and down with excitement. Why? Because most of my calls come from advertising agencies requesting models to promote hospitals, banks, insurance companies, etc. Get the idea? They need real people. Now, do you see why I get so excited? These people usually don't even realize the opportunities in the modeling business. They don't sit around, about to celebrate their 50th birthday and decide, "Hey, I think I should be a model." Everyone assumes you have to be 5'9", thin and beautiful to be a model. It is just not true. You'll learn a lot more about the subject when you get to Character Modeling in Chapter 6.

I get excited about all kinds of people because I need all kinds of people to make my agency work. Most agencies have the same needs that mine does. Only the largest markets have a great demand for high-fashion models.

My agency is not a school, but I offer a one-time training session. This is to polish the people who have no clue about being a professional model and/or the modeling business. You need to know something! When I send someone to see a potential client, I want to feel confident she/he will make a good impression of herself/himself as well as my agency.

An agency is responsible for every aspect of promoting a model's career — from collecting your monetary compensation, to scheduling your time, to simply keeping you updated and fashionable in the current market. It is your job to prove that they should invest in you instead of the many other models who may be equally qualified on a physical level. At the end of this section, you will find a sample of a modeling resume'/outline. Have photos and a resume' available at every modeling interview. I have included this information to give you some advance preparation for knowing agency procedures and expectations.

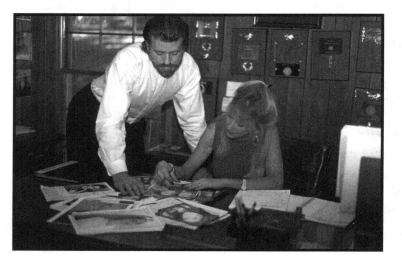

Marsha at work with her husband, Dean. Photographer: Mark Hanson

Many models who have not attended a school have gone directly into modeling through an agency. You must have pictures to successfully represent yourself to an agency. Snapshots are fine. For high fashion, you should have a good head shot wearing very little makeup and your hair pulled away from your face. You should also include a full-length body shot wearing a leotard or swimsuit. Your pictures should be of good clarity, with your height, weight, bust, waist and hip measurements written on the back. Know exactly, to the quarter inch, all of your measurements. Remember, be honest. An agency will know when you walk in the door if you have lied about your measurements. Include your name and telephone number on the back of all photos. If you're planning to target agencies in a large market, don't waste your money on professional photographs. An agency that is interested in you will set up test shots with their hairstylists, makeup artists and photographers. If an agency thinks you have tremendous potential, you may be signed immediately. Many people have become professional models with little or no school training or modeling experience.

A big agency will expect you to learn the basics quickly. Then they will put your knowledge to work for you. Even if you have never modeled before, if you look good in your "test shots," an agency may want to work with you. Agencies exist to represent models and to find jobs for them. You should examine carefully any agency with which you expect to work. The reputation of a modeling agency may be easier to determine than that of a modeling school. Ask other models who have aspired to goals similar to your own, and listen carefully to people you trust when they express their opinions and tell their stories about how they got started.

If you are in a small to medium size city, you will want to have some professional pictures to show. That makes it easier for agencies like mine to market you. Currently many agencies use laser (color) copies, instead of original photographs, which makes it much less expensive for the model. The cost of the copies from an original negative is about $1.25 to $2.00 per copy. My clients usually hire models based solely on their laser copies. Pictures are essential in the modeling business.

Before visiting an agency, call ahead and find out when they interview. If you arrive completely prepared, you will appear more professional. Be prompt, courteous, and by all means, don't offer excuses if you are late — just prove that you can perform despite the odds. Answer all questions clearly and intelligently, and thank your interviewer before you leave. Remember, it is possible to turn heads by making the correct first impression.

You may think that during your first visit to an agency you should dress in trendy fashions in order to catch your interviewer's attention immediately. Advantageous as it may seem, you should not project an image that is unnatural or affected. Catch your interviewer's attention with the "you" that you are! Dress in a way that expresses your sense of style, but avoid wearing baggy or loose-fitting clothes. Agencies want to see the shape of your body. Don't be shy. Remember, you are promoting your looks, which includes your body, as well as your face. Also avoid excessive makeup, hair spray and anything else that will distract from your natural look. Although everyone's sense of the modeling business involves glamour and sophistication, most modeling agencies will want to see what you have to offer without any artificial enhancements. Your "natural look" will be the one that appeals to them the most during the initial visit.

If you are turned away for whatever reason, remember that it may not necessarily have to do with you directly. Models are commonly rejected, either because they don't have the look that the agency is seeking, or sometimes an agency may have too many models who already have a "look" similar to yours. Whatever the case, you must be willing to try again. Essentially, timing is everything. So visit another agency as soon as you can.

You should visit as many agencies as possible during the amount of time that you have set aside for "open calling" (personally calling on agencies in a professional manner). Because rejection is a part of all modeling careers, plan for it. As I mentioned earlier, you should not become discouraged when you are turned away from a particular agency or assignment. In a career that focuses almost entirely on appearance, you must be able to accept criticism with grace, perseverance and determination. Remember that every modeling agency is unique. Each person with whom you interview is likely to admire different traits and features. Different agencies will seek different "looks." Though rejection is common in the modeling business, your chances of discovery will improve with each person you meet.

You may become very discouraged when an interviewer looks at your photograph for a few seconds, then looks at you and says, "Forget it! We're not interested." How, in less than a minute, can they make a decision? Agencies are in the business of shopping for people. They shop for specific looks and types. Just as you shop for clothes, they shop for people. And just like you can flip through a clothes rack in a few seconds, they can flip through a "rack" of people with similar speed! An agency may seem like they're brushing you off, but they're not — interviewers know what they need when they see it!

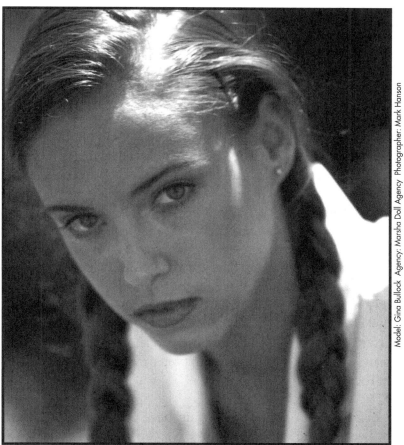

Model: Gina Bullock Agency: Marsha Doll Agency Photographer: Mark Hanson

While it is impossible to separate rejection from the modeling industry, many people will eventually achieve success. Keep this in mind, especially when you feel like retiring to a different line of work. Nearly every model has been rejected for some type of assignment. You will probably experience more rejection than acceptance in the world of modeling. Use your determination to your advantage and refuse to accept failure. You will find that more opportunities will arise. The real advantage is you will emerge a stronger, more capable person and a better model!

When I meet a person who is interested in this business, the first thing I say is, "This business is tough." If I think someone truly has a "look", then I try to evaluate him or her mentally and emotionally. Can she handle being away from home? How about all of the rejection involved in this business? Is he dedicated and professional? If I believe the answers to these three questions are yes, that's when I try to place him or her with an agency in a big city, like New York. To do this, I simply take a couple of snapshots (head and full length) and send them to the agencies. If the person is accepted, I am considered the "Mother Agency" and receive a five percent commission on everything the model makes. That commission is taken from the agency, not the model. Now, I know your next question is, "Do I need a Mother Agency?" The answer is, no, not necessarily. My agency is a reputable business, and I have made many "connections" with influential agencies worldwide. Maybe they take my opinion of a model more seriously than other small-town agencies. But who knows? I personally believe from my experience as an agent, that models have a better chance to succeed when they understand the nature of the business. It is my responsibility to prepare my models before sending them off to the "Big City."

Though some of the models I train have great potential, they go undiscovered for quite some time. For example, Steve was a blue-collar worker from a small town who had no real experience when I first met him. We worked steadily for several months, and he rapidly improved his skills and enhanced his modeling abilities. We made the rounds to the agencies, but they just weren't interested in him. In fact, Steve was discouraged about his prospects and was considering giving up on modeling altogether. But he didn't. After trying for several years, Steve was chosen by an agency to model in Paris. He was then asked to travel to many different countries, where he became a successful and highly sought after professional model. To date, he has modeled professionally all over Europe! Very often, as in Steve's case, models who don't sign with an agency in the United States travel to Europe where they can prepare for international modeling and the rigorous requirements of big American cities like New York.

Like Steve, Angie is another model who wasn't immediately recognized for her potential. Because Angie had personal problems, I was hoping that modeling would give her some direction in life. She had a real "tomboyish" nature that was very appealing, and I thought her look would be a refreshing change for the industry. So we worked carefully on polishing her skills. Angie went "open calling" to every agency she could find. Like most hopeful models, she experienced numerous rejections. She also had to accept criticism from various agency directors who suggested that she should lose 15 pounds before they would be interested in her. She refused to give up and followed the agency directors' advice. She lost the weight and returned to sign with a prestigious agency that had turned her away before. After working successfully in Paris for two years, she worked in New York City for several more and carved out her own niche as an ambitious, committed professional model.

Let's get back to your search for an agency to represent you. You have your pictures, you've gone on a few interviews, and an agency "wants" you. What next? Do not immediately sign with the first agency that seems interested in you. Though you will be anxious to get started, you have time to "shop around" and decide which agency will best represent you (and vice versa, of course). This can be one of the biggest, most crucial decisions you will ever make. If you know you are good enough to sign with at least one agency, remind yourself of this: perhaps others will be interested in you, too! The list of agencies in the back of this publication will make you aware of the many opportunities you have.

You may be required to sign a contract before you can work for an agency. First, you should confirm the agency's credibility on a national level. Though signing contracts is not an unusual thing to do, you need to exercise caution before you jump into such a transaction. Some agencies don't require models to sign contracts before they allow them to work, but you will find that most agencies do want their models to sign a contract of some sort. Be certain that you feel completely comfortable with the terms and conditions that will be required of you. NEVER sign anything without reading it completely.

Before you give an agency exclusive rights to represent you, make sure there is enough work for you to do for that particular agency. If you sign a contract and assignments become less frequent, you will be in a bad position. You will have committed yourself to a company that can't provide everything you need — and basically, you will be trapped! So, again, know exactly what you are getting into.

Sample Agency Resume'

Use the sample resume' on the following page to prepare your own resume' for trips to modeling/ talent agencies. The example includes some general guidelines. You can change the order or types of categories to express your characteristics and experience in the most effective way. No matter how you choose to prepare the categories, be sure to type them neatly on clean, professional-looking paper. This is just an example to show you what the agencies will find interesting about you. Always attach your resume' on the back of your 8x10 black and white head shot if you are targeting talent agencies. Make sure the size of your resume' is the same size as the photograph. This makes the agent's job easier when it comes to filing potential models. If you are targeting modeling agencies, a resume' is not as important. What modeling agencies want are snapshots with your height, weight and age written on the back.

Sarah Haley
100 Oak Street
Centerville, U.S.A..
Date Of Birth: April 10, 1982
Physical Characteristics:
Height 5'9"   Hair Color — Brunette
Weight 120 pounds   Complexion Shade — Medium
Bust — 34 inches   Shoe Size/Width — 9M
Waist — 25 inches   Clothing Size — 7
Hips — 35 inches   Eye Color — Green

• Educational background: Currently attending Florida
  State University, Major: communications

• Modeling/ Acting school(s) attended: Currently en-
  rolled as a student in Karen's School for Models,
  Centerville, U.S.A.; two years at the FSU School of
  Theater.

* Modeling/ Acting Experience: Participated in several
  local fashion shows; runway experience; television
  experience; lead role in two university lab plays.

Titles/Honors Achieved: Placed lst in the Runway Competition and placed 2nd in the Television Commercial
Competition at the Models of the South Convention in
1997.

Union Affiliation: Member, American Federation of
Television and Radio Artists.

(*Give specific details)

Freelance Modeling

Believe it or not, some models do not strive for single-agency representation! This is most prevalent in small to medium markets. Freelance models go door-to-door looking for work on their own. Some work for several different agencies at the same time without being bound by a particular contract. You may be surprised to know that some models prefer this type of modeling. Single-agency representation has the obvious advantage of having someone who will find the best assignments for you. Freelance models have the advantage of having "no strings attached." They don't have contract restrictions, can make their own choices and can essentially create their own careers.

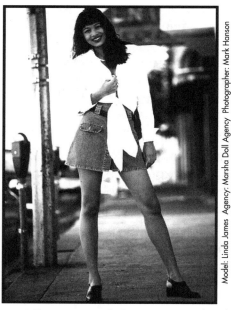

Model: Linda James Agency: Marsha Doll Agency Photographer: Mark Hanson

Though it sounds intimidating, freelance modeling offers some benefits — you are the deciding factor when it comes to choosing an assignment. This is challenging work, but if you are the type of person who likes to take on your own responsibilities, it may hold some promise for you.

Weigh carefully the advantages and disadvantages of your own situation: Do you need extra guidance when it comes to business matters? Do you need that extra push when it comes to keeping regular work hours? If so, you may need the extra support that one agency can provide. But if none of these questions applies to you, you may be a candidate for becoming a freelance model.

If you are represented by one agency and under contract with them, obviously they are going to watch over you and your decisions carefully, but they may not have enough work. Also, your agency may not give you the exposure you need. As a freelance model, you are free to work for whomever you choose — the options are endless! Men and women who are assertive and independent can meet this challenge and make it work for them. I do recommend, however, that you start out with an agency first, rather than trying to model without any kind of guidance. If you work with an agency first, you will become more familiar with the booking procedures and the business aspects of modeling. After you have acquired this knowledge, you will be in a better position to manage your own career. If you choose to freelance, it is possible to work with several agencies in the small to medium markets. In a large market, however, an agent is a necessity. So choose one carefully. There are only a handful out there that make a difference in the world of modeling.

Chapter 2
Modeling
Characteristics

CHAPTER 2

MODELING CHARACTERISTICS

Your Personality

Because modeling is a stressful and sometimes disheartening pro-fession, you may find that you are not always able to project in-credible degrees of enthusiasm at every given moment. Everyone has that problem, no matter what the career. It would be unrea-sonable for me to suggest that you must always smile gracefully and be totally agreeable when you are being criticized by someone you just met. But it is always bad business to act defensively or belligerently toward others.

Accepting the opinions of others is an important quality that a model must practice. There will always be agents and directors who insist that you must change your hair, your weight, and vari-ous other things. One agency may tell you that you need to cut your hair. Another will tell you they like it long. If you seriously intend to work with an agency, and you strongly believe a sugges-tion is in your best interest, take the advice. Whether it is to lose weight or to change your hairstyle, do it — if you think it will make a difference to you and your career.

Following an agency's advice is a great way to make an impression. It will be harder for an agent to criticize your look after you have done exactly what he's asked! No one likes to receive criticism, but certain people are admired for handling it better than others — you want to be one of those people.

Act like a mature, reasonable adult in each and every situation. You will undoubtedly impress those with whom you are interview-ing or working. You must always act like you love what you do, because pretty faces can be found anywhere. "Pretty" personalities are scarce. If you aren't pleasing your clients or your agent(s), a replacement is easy to find! No matter how you are feeling, you must project maturity, dedication and a good attitude.

Physical Characteristics of a Model

Most sought-after, high-fashion female models range in height from 5'9" and up. These models are tall and thin, with a statuesque appearance, and their ages generally range from 14-23 years old. Petite models range from 5'3" to 5'8" in height. There is also a growing demand for oversized (or "plus-size") models. These models typically wear clothing sizes 10-20, and range in height from 5'9" and up.

Most importantly, female high-fashion models must have beautiful, well-defined legs, with kneecaps that are placed high above the ankles. Female models are also expected to have good, clear skin; well-defined eyes; neatly-cut, stylish hair; and correct posture.

Male fashion models need to have the following physical characteristics: they should wear jacket size 40-42; have a 30"-34" waist; a 40"-42" chest; and a size 15"-17" neck. They should range in height from 6' to 6'2 1/2", and they must try to maintain a weight of 155-180 pounds, depending on their height. Obviously, these men should also have well-groomed hair, a clear complexion and proper posture.

Every agency has different height requirements, so call before you go on an interview to make sure your visit won't be a waste of your valuable time. As brutal as it may seem, an agency will not interview you unless you meet their minimum height standard! Many men and women have been disappointed to learn that their height can prevent them from getting an interview.

The above standards are suggested characteristics for high-fashion models. Don't be discouraged if you feel you are lacking in some of these requirements. Height is the main requirement that is "set in stone" by each particular agency. You may have some latitude in the other categories.

As I mentioned earlier, you must work diligently to become a model, and if you don't try, you will never know your capabilities. If a modeling agency recommends some things you should change about yourself in order to work for them, I suggest that you give it a try. Once you have lost a little weight or changed your hairstyle, go back and prove that you are committed and willing to do what's necessary to become a model. However, don't do anything that makes you feel uncomfortable. What one agency tells you to do may be the opposite of what another one wants! Only make changes to your look if you think you can handle the "new you." It is also important to remember that character models (a topic which will be covered in Chapter 6) represent "real-life" people. If you cannot become a high-fashion model, you may still have another opportunity awaiting you!

A Basic Wardrobe for Models

On rare occasions, models may have to provide some elements of their own wardrobes to accentuate their appearance while on certain assignments. However, providing your own wardrobe is not a common practice in a large modeling market. If you are from a smaller city, you may have to provide your own clothing on occasion. Although your clothing is usually provided by your client, you may be asked at the last minute to bring along specific accessories or outfits to a job site. If this happens, you don't want to have your best clothing unavailable, dirty or torn. Be prepared and plan ahead.

Consider carrying a small bag to hold your basic jewelry, like a strand of pearls, some gold or silver earrings and similar items. Don't take any trendy accessories along. Chances are slim that they will match your outfit. Do take along some of your favorite, classically simple accessories. Learn to keep your possessions in excellent condition. Keep your wardrobe clean, pressed and on hangers at all times. If you are borrowing someone else's clothing (either a friend's or a store owner's) always return the items in good shape, so you may borrow them on other occasions, should you need to.

As an aspiring model, there are certain types of basic clothing you may want to have in abundance. Look for plain, interesting colors. Black and white do not photograph well for most models. Avoid large, loud prints that will distract from your beauty in a picture or on film. Seek interesting textures like suede or leather — they make for a more exciting picture. Use your common sense when choosing your wardrobe. And remember, try to always keep your best clothing ready for action and choose basic styles that can be used often!

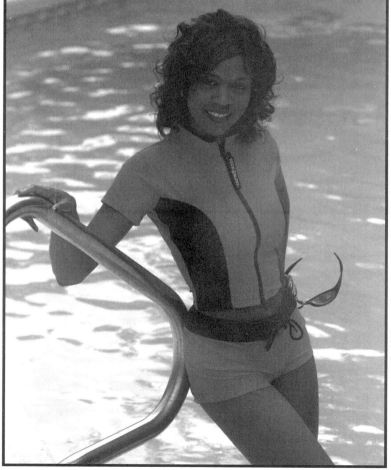

Model: Kenyetta Close Agency: Marsha Doll Agency Photographer: Phil Coale

Chapter 3
Photographers & Portfolios

PHOTOGRAPHERS & PORTFOLIOS

Working With Photographers

As I mentioned previously, many models gain valuable experience without ever attending a modeling school. This usually involves working diligently on their own to create a portfolio or a "book" that will appear professionally crafted. Contrary to what you may believe, creating a portfolio and developing working relationships with various photographers do not have to involve large sums of money. You can get the

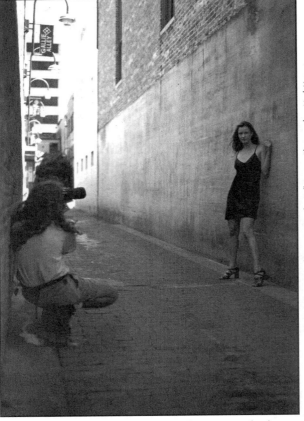

Model: Michelle Harwood Agency: Marsha Doll Agency Photographer: Mark Hanson

pictures you need simply being careful, making good choices, and by being a discriminating subject. A photographer may use you as a subject to compile his own portfolio, in return for some pictures that you can keep. If you're in a large market, having a book is not necessary to find representation, just snapshots. If an agency likes your look, they will want to do their own testing. In small to medium markets where photographers and jobs are limited, agencies usually prefer you already have several professional photographs. It makes it easier for them to get you jobs.

Much like choosing an agency or a school, you do not have to settle for working with the first photographer you meet. You can afford to be choosy when making major career decisions, and you will not be sorry later for doing so! When a photographer approaches you, check his or her references with the Better Business Bureau or with another reliable source before agreeing to pose for any photographs. Even after you have carefully inspected a photographer's referrals, it may be wise to take someone along with you during your initial visit to his or her home or office. Avoid a potentially dangerous situation. Take a friend along for moral support!

Many photographers are looking for new models in order to provide the modeling industry with contemporary and exciting new faces. They could possibly employ you to increase their own professional portfolios. From this, you may be able to gain print jobs that will further develop your portfolio for presentation to agencies or clients. Besides training you to pose in front of a camera, the photographer may be able to give you terrific exposure in fashion magazines, newspapers and, possibly, catalogs, depending upon his own abilities, connections, and reputation.

Always remember that every photographer may be a future contact for employment. Try to be prompt, optimistic and enthusiastic, even on your worst day. In retrospect, your attitude may be what they remember most about you, and it may determine how willing they are to assist you at other times.

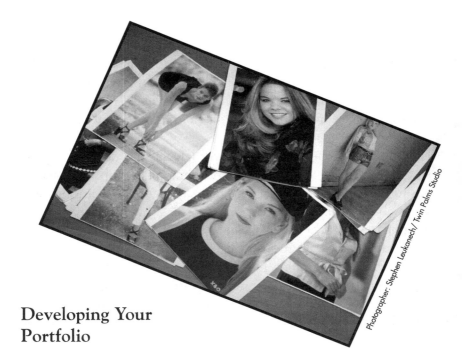

Developing Your Portfolio

Your portfolio is your most important promotional tool. You will compile a portfolio as you progress through your modeling career. This is called your "book." It should contain your tear sheets (advertisements and editorials that have previously appeared in magazines, catalogs or newspapers) and your most impressive 8" x 10" photographs. These photographs can be color or black and white, and they should include a good variety of "head shots" and "full-length shots," along with your name, your address and the name of your agency. Versatility is a crucial factor in determining which pictures to use. Try to "sell yourself" by displaying a variety of different looks in order to interest all potential clients. Your agency should have the expertise to do this for you. While the content of your book is not restricted in terms of creativity, it is imperative to include <u>only</u> your best photographs. To include mediocre shots will decrease both the value and the impact of the final product. Keep your book full of current shots at all times. This will show agency directors and clients that you are actively involved in modeling. A book full of old pictures only proves that you have not been very motivated about updating either your appearance or your performance.

Once you are listed with an agency, your book is invaluable. Many times a client will call several different agencies, looking for a particular type of model for a job. The agencies send their models' books to the client who makes selections based solely on photographs. Do you see how important your book is?

Even before you have completed enough print work to assemble a book (especially when you are first starting out in a small market),

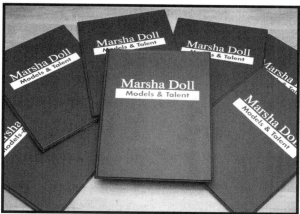

you will find it necessary to have two or three excellent pictures of yourself readily available for inspection. Keep these photographs in your possession at all times, particularly when interviewing with an agency. When the directors ask for your pictures, you must have them organized and ready for presentation. You should always be able to provide interviewers with at least two pictures of yourself, a head shot and full length. Your biggest mistake would be to go through any door without your pictures. Any model who walks in without pictures won't get much consideration. Modeling is essentially about marketing your assets, and no one wants to invest in a model without knowing his or her photographic qualities. So, go ahead! Use your pictures to your advantage.

It could require a great deal of time and money to travel to the cities where modeling is prevalent and profitable. Some modeling candidates may not have the available resources to travel directly to such model markets as New York, Los Angeles or Miami. Therefore, I suggest that you send your snapshots with a well-written cover letter to the people with whom you'd like to meet, whether they are school instructors, agency directors, photographers or producers. Because agencies and schools receive a great deal of mail, you shouldn't expect to have these pictures returned to you, unless you specify this in your letter and include a self-addressed, stamped envelope. Even then, they may be too involved in their business dealings to send your pictures back to you. So, it's best to send your pictures after you've had copies made.

You may use the sample letter enclosed in this book or you may choose to write something that reflects your personal style. The list at the end of this book will give you some potential starting points for places to send these letters and pictures. Whatever you write, make it brief, honest and grammatically correct. Include your age, height, weight, hair and eye color, and the time and place where you can be reached.

This type of correspondence, though not always answered immediately, may generate some very positive results. But for this to happen, you should try to make your letter look as professional and as carefully crafted as possible. Always call ahead and obtain the exact name (spelling included) of the person who will be receiving your letter. Ask for the person in charge of "New Faces." This will ensure that your letter reaches its destination and will show that you took the time to address your letter properly.

(Sample Letter)

Today's Date

Ms. First M. Last
Title of Person
Name of Agency
555 Center Street Address
New York, New York 10010

Dear Ms. Last:

I am very interested in pursuing a modeling career and have enclosed some photographs for your review.

I am currently sixteen years old. My height is 5 feet, 8 inches, and I weigh 115 pounds. I would appreciate having the opportunity to visit you for a brief interview and can be reached daily at my home telephone number after 4:30 p.m. Thank you for your consideration. I look forward to your response.

Sincerely yours,

Sarah Haley
2995 South Grove Street
Main City, Utah 00000
123/456-7890

Chapter 4
Composites

COMPOSITES

A Model's Business Card

A composite, also referred to as your "comp", is usually an 8" x 6" card (although the size can vary) that serves as a business card for a professional model. Much like your pictures, composites are essential for communicating your vital statistics to the world. Your composite will include your best pictures, the name of your agency, your union affiliation (if you are a member of either AFTRA or SAG), your telephone number and address, your hair and eye color and all of your basic measurements — height, weight, bust, waist, hips, clothing size and shoe size.

You most likely will be presenting these cards to interested photographers and agency directors who are interested in seeing your versatility. Your statistics and a "head shot" (also called a "beauty shot") usually go on the front of the card. Remember to include several different pictures with varying poses on the back of the card. You don't have to be restricted to a front/back format on your card (see next paragraph). Just be sure to include a wide variety of pictures! While these pictures can be either black and white or color, make sure they are exciting shots that display you at your very best. (If money is an issue, black and white photographs will serve the purpose very well.) As your career in modeling progresses, you will want your composite to portray your creativity and your versatility.

Composite Format

You don't have to confine yourself to a specific format for your composites. You will be surprised to see a number of different styles and types of composites: some combine black and white with color photography; some have several pages that fold out; and some have photos on the front and back of a one-page card.

Since your composite is your "business card," it should be as exciting and versatile as possible. Let your agency compile your best work for your composite. It should look slick, like an advertisement. In fact, it is an advertisement — for you.

The construction of your composite should be left up to your agent or someone you trust in the business. Avoid spending a lot of money on composites — the most important thing to express is your beauty, your ability to photograph well and your individuality. If you're in a small market, composites are not necessary. Don't waste your money. Watch out for people who will try to take advantage of you by convincing you to spend a fortune on your composite. This is an another example of where you can spend a moderate amount of money and still have a good product.

Many prospective clients, photographers and agency directors will look at your composite as a direct reflection of you and your abilities. Keep several available at all times. Be proud to present them — a composite proves you have a professional edge!

Chapter 5
Motion Pictures, Pageants, Fashion Show Hints, Trade Shows

Chapter 5

Motion Pictures, Pageants, Fashion Show Hints, & Trade Shows

Becoming an "Extra"

Landing a part as an "extra" in a motion picture can be a very exciting experience for someone who is just becoming familiar with film production. Being "behind the scenes" on a movie set will give you a new appreciation for the hard work and the commitment involved in film making. While the pay isn't very high for movie "extras", you will gain some critical insight into the acting industry.

Many people consider their modeling careers to be stepping stones to future careers in acting. Sometimes, this can have advantages, because you are "experienced" in film production, but some film producers don't like to work with people who claim to be aspiring models. So, trying to break into acting with a modeling background may be more difficult than if you just walked into a film audition off the street.

With some degree of luck and confidence in your abilities, you may be one of the people who gets promoted to a small principal role in a film. This is some of the best exposure you will get. Check with the office of your local film commissioner or your local Chamber of Commerce. If any films are planned in your vicinity, they will know about them and can give you the necessary details. Another way to prepare for future film auditions is to leave some of your current pictures at a local agency or modeling school because "extras" often are discovered this way. Exposure is not the only advantage of appearing in a motion picture — credible careers in both modeling and acting can be the end result.

On the subject of films, it's important that we discuss union affiliation. You may already be, or you may aspire to be, associated with either the Screen Actors' Guild (SAG) or the American Federation of Television and Radio Artists (AFTRA). To become a union member, you will have to meet several requirements. When you officially become a member of SAG or AFTRA, you are immediately considered a "professional", and film producers will be required to pay you a higher amount than they would a typical "extra." Naturally, your professional acting status could prevent you from acquiring small acting roles, because the producers will not necessarily want to pay more money for your services. As you can see, there are advantages and disadvantages to being affiliated with unions. Personally, I suggest doing everything you can to acquire a SAG or an AFTRA card or both. It is a sign that you have film experience, and your union affiliation should be listed on your applications to agencies and on your composites.

Participating in Beauty Pageants

A beauty pageant can be an another tool to assist you in gaining confidence for a future modeling career. However, like film production, no pageant will be able to help you achieve overnight success as an international model — especially not the smaller, less prestigious ones. Pageants are helpful in terms of what they teach you about the psychological aspects of competition. A pageant is the classic example of the ultimate in rejection — 50 girls may be competing in the contest, but only one of them will go home as the first-place winner. The same is true of modeling for many people, as the odds are precisely that high. In a pageant, you will be competing against hundreds of beautiful girls, many of whom have the exact same qualifications you do. A pageant can help you with three important objectives: 1) You will learn more about how to stand out in a crowd and how to set yourself apart from those around you; 2) You will learn that rejection really exists; and 3) You will probably learn how to deal with the stress that rejection causes. Valuable experience like this will truly be to your advantage when you begin to model. If such an opportunity comes your way, and if you have nothing to lose, I suggest that you try to compete.

Don't enter a pageant only with the intention of becoming the next Miss Teen U.S.A. See what you can learn from the behind-the-scenes events. Learn how to be confident in front of a large audience. Practice having a good attitude despite the circumstances. Put yourself in situations where you may be discovered! A pageant may provide you with the visibility to make that possible. You never know who may be watching!

Most of all, turn a pageant into a chance for you to build a foundation for the modeling world. Concentrate specifically on the large, highly advertised pageants to make certain that the information and skills you're learning are universal. The *Miss Watermelon Patch Pageant* probably won't be first on the list of an agent who's looking for fresh talent.

Participating in Fashion Shows

Fashion shows in small to medium markets can be another terrific opportunity to show the world your poise and your confidence! Generally, your participation in fashion shows will be arranged by your school or agency, but if you are asked to participate in one by a friend or another reliable source (and if you feel comfortable with the procedures), you might find it to your advantage to accept the invitation. Again, this is a great way to gain experience and self-confidence.

Because the fashion show garments typically will be loaned to you by trendy boutiques or store owners, keep them in good condition, as if they were your own. Avoid getting makeup, cologne or deodorant stains (you should wear unscented deodorant only) on borrowed clothing. Otherwise, you risk creating problems for yourself or the person responsible for the fashion show. Be sure to use care when dressing and undressing. Putting a scarf over your head before pulling on your shirts, dresses or other garments will prevent any unnecessary stains or unsightly marks. Returning the clothing to hangers and boxes when you have finished with them will prolong their "life expectancies" and will ensure that the store owner won't be hesitant to loan you clothes on another occasion.

While a fashion show is in progress, you may find yourself back-stage with several different people who are frantically trying to look appropriately dressed. Behind the scenes at a fashion show can be a hectic place to be, but don't let it get the best of you. Follow these few, simple rules that will help you "fit in" with the rest of the crowd:

1) Don't chew gum, eat, drink or smoke during a fashion show, even when you are out of view. Not only may this jeopardize the condition of your garments, but it may also be offensive to the people around you. Don't sit down in your fashion show garments, because they may wrinkle. No one likes to make last minute changes for any reason!

2) Be sure that tags and labels do not stick out of your clothing. Tuck them neatly in your waistband or in your sleeves, or remove and save them to be replaced after the show.

3) Do not object to any outfit that you are asked to wear. This will upset the organization of the show and will limit your future invitations to other shows. The clothes that you wear are generally at the discretion of the designer or the coordinator of the program, and they do not have the time or the patience to deal with attitude problems. Remember to act like you always love your job!

4) Report the damage of a garment immediately to whomever is in charge of the show. It is your responsibility to make sure the clothes are in their best condition before you put them on.

5) Report to fashion shows on time and neatly dressed. Also, don't leave your dressing room after you have arrived for the show. You never know when you might be needed.

Trade Show and Convention Bookings

Many convention directors or manufacturers hire models to enhance a particular product, for example, an automobile or a boat, by having models stand next to the item. These models will also give prospective buyers information that may influence them to make a purchase. At these all-day shows, the manufacturer hopes to sell as many products as possible. Generally, trade show models must be attractive, and they must be able to interact with people (the customers) by presenting a delightful and witty personality at a moment's notice.

While a modeling job of this type seems simple to do, the model must be able to answer questions about the product he or she is demonstrating. The model must also be prepared to hand out samples while engaged in conversation. Trade show models will rely primarily on their abilities to charm the public, as they act somewhat like salespeople. A real salesperson will be available, but the models often must entertain the customers until the salesperson is able to help them personally. Nearly every model has participated in this type of modeling and has gained an appreciation for learning how to be a "selling point" of a product.

The most prestigious position for a trade show model is the classification of model spokesperson. This person must be qualified to speak comfortably about the product or the company responsible for the show. If you have an aptitude for speaking and writing, you should attempt to gain such a position. These models are in high demand!

Trade shows are typically held in hotels or convention centers, and they are not always open to the public. Very often, the customers will be retailers representing large store chains, and they will be buying the products for sale in bulk quantities only, so the general public usually does not attend. Medical shows, pharmaceutical shows, home appliance shows, toy shows and cosmetology shows represent the types of shows usually closed to the public. Those open to the public may include flower shows, automobile shows and boat shows. At either type of show, the model's duties are the same: display the product; demonstrate the product, if necessary; answer questions; be helpful; and be courteous!

Since the town where my agency is located is not considered high fashion, my models receive a lot of promotional work. The pay for promotional jobs ranges from $10 to $25 per hour. Even though these opportunities don't pay as well as other modeling jobs, the same level of professionalism is still expected. Promotions are an excellent opportunity for a model to display responsibility and enthusiasm. It's just not that hard to be punctual, smile and have a good a time with whatever you're promoting. Some promotions last for weeks or even months. After a while, some models become complacent and are replaced. Every model starts somewhere. Enjoy what you do, or someone else will.

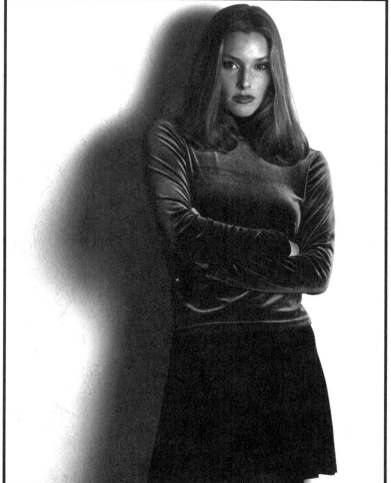

Model: Emily Fletcher Agency: Marsha Doll Agency Photographer: Stephen Leukanech/ Twin Palms Studio

Chapter 6
Character, Child, Plus, Petite, Specialty & Male Models

CHARACTER, CHILD, PLUS, PETITE, SPECIALTY & MALE MODELS

Characteristics of Character Models

Character models represent "real-life" people — people that you see in everyday situations. Because television and print commercials require people from different backgrounds who can appear to be "typical" housewives, businessmen, parents or other such common figures, character models are in great demand. Many advertisements require infants, children, young adults, middle-aged people or senior citizens as models in order to make the advertisement as effective as possible. Advertising agencies and production companies want to create a commercial or an advertisement to which the public will easily relate. They hire models who look like ordinary people, with the intention of selling an idea or a product.

Think about a commercial you have recently seen. Didn't that woman selling diapers look like your idea of a new mother? And the older, more mature man who appeared in the commercial for vitamins — didn't he remind you of your own dad or grandfather? Character models are used for just that reason. They are supposed to attract customers for their clients, so the idea that every model must be a heart-stopping beauty is not always valid. Traditionally, beautiful models promote beauty products. That's because we all tend to believe that the lipstick Cindy Crawford is wearing is going to look as good on us as it does on her. And you know what? It sells! We all want to look better. So when you see a beautiful person advertising something, the message is that the product will make us as beautiful. That's the reason for the people behind the products. I can't tell you the number of lipsticks I own — and my lips are still thin!

If it's not a beauty product that's being marketed, more than likely you'll see "real people" in the advertisements. Modeling is not always about being beautiful; it's about selling products. Have you ever seen a gorgeous blonde in an advertisement for house-

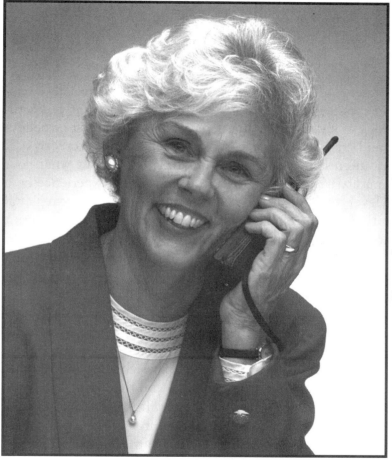

Model: Jo Ann Dull Agency: Marsha Doll Agency
Photographer: Stephen Leukanech/ Twin Palms Studio

hold cleaners or mildew remover? You probably haven't, simply because the general public expects those products to be used by a middle-aged housewife. It's an unfair presumption, but it's true! Any company, agency or business with an "ordinary" product like bleach to sell doesn't want to intimidate the public by using glamorous figures in their ads; rather, they attempt to make the public relate to their product by showing ordinary-looking "house-wives" using it.

In other words, there are no limits to the definition of a character model. There is a great demand for normal, stereotypical people. Look at a bug spray ad in any magazine. Watch the television commercial for pizza. Who do you see? You see character models. And they have just as good of a chance for a successful modeling career as do models in high fashion. And the career of a successful character model will traditionally outlive the careers of most high-fashion models.

Character modeling requires some acting ability, especially if television commercials are your goal. It's important that you actually look as if you belong in the picture, and you must be believable and credible in your portrayal of a particular stereotype. If you're interested in character modeling, check out what your community has to offer. After acquiring acting experience on a local level (including theater, commercials, etc.), pursue regional opportunities. As your acting experience advances, you may want to target a larger market. At that time, you may be required to produce a black and white head shot and a resume of your acting experience. It may also be a good time to find an agency to represent your acting career.

Agencies that represent character/commercial-type models are called talent agencies. The larger the market, the greater importance will be placed on your acting experience. A full resume, listing diverse amounts of commercial and theatrical skills, will be essential for promoting your talents. If you have no experience for your resume, I suggest you get involved on a local/regional level. Take some acting classes. Learn how to do a professional audition in front of a camera. Get involved with companies that perform plays in your community.

If acting is not for you, print modeling may be the opportunity you're looking for. Models are selected based upon their photos, instead of their auditioning skills. Still, the greatest possibilities present themselves to the model who is the most versatile. Be prepared for all of it.

Child Models — Who is a Candidate?

Young people are typically involved in character modeling, but it is not unusual to see children involved in various other types of modeling careers. Although exceptionally beautiful children may have a better chance of becoming fashion models, a child model does not require perfect features to become successful. (It is essential, however, that they are somewhat patient and well behaved.) Like adult character models, a child with average looks has a good chance of becoming the center of a television advertisement that represents all of America's children. His or her personality and level of confidence is the key?

Be forewarned, however, that modeling is often more difficult for children. Modeling can stress a child's happiness and mental health, much more than it would an adult. Children usually have delightful and innocent demeanors, and because they have more

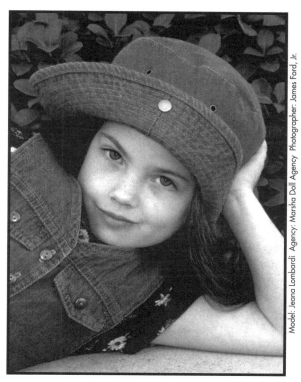

Model: Jeana Lombardi Agency: Marsha Doll Agency Photographer: James Ford, Jr.

difficulty expressing themselves, many parents don't realize when they are putting too much responsibility on a youngster. Because child modeling is exciting for parents (It's great to see potential at such a young age!), some parents get carried away with promoting their children's talent. This can create problems.

If your child is totally receptive to the idea of modeling, then great opportunities may arise. Just be certain you remember that children are delicate — they are not miniature adults. A child's attention span is incredibly short. Ambition is the last thing on a child's mind. Don't try to force them to model, because they will not have the same dedication to modeling as do adults.

Child modeling can be very expensive if you do not live in a large market area. Agencies often use child models who live within their market so the child is available at a moment's notice for appointments, auditions and interviews. But what if an agency in New

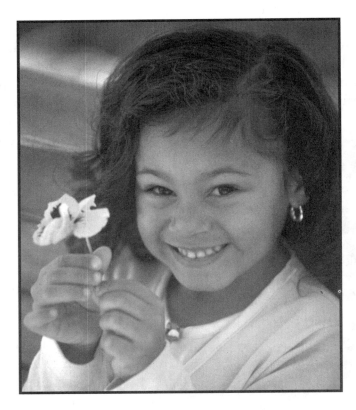

Model: Jazmine Harper. Agency: Marsha Doll Agency
Photographer: Mark Hanson

York wants to sign your child, and your family lives in Colorado? Arrangements between you and the agency will be made. The most common situation entails you living in New York during the summer months and during the holidays. This can be expensive, especially if you're going on interviews everyday, with few results. Many times you will experience this kind of pain when you are first starting out.

So, if you and your child live in a remote area of the country, plan to wait until your child matures and is able to show a real commitment to modeling; otherwise you may spend more money than necessary, and you probably won't get your anticipated results.

If you live near large cities like New York or Chicago, it may be worth your time to take your child in to interview with a modeling or talent agency. Of course, your child will need to have some good snapshots taken for review by the agencies you plan to visit. As with adult models, you should not plan to invest in a great number of pictures. An agency representative will be able to tell from some basic snapshots if your child has modeling capabilities. Also, have a song or monologue prepared in case the agent asks your child to perform. This will be a great opportunity for them to see your child's talent and personality.

Many agencies specialize in child modeling, so call ahead and schedule some interviews! As you go through the interviewing process, however, remember to have your child's pictures updated frequently. Children's features change drastically in a short period of time, and it is important to have current pictures that portray them as they are at that very moment.

Many models are young when they begin their careers. Have you ever considered why this may be? Many famous high-fashion models are 14, 15 and 16 years old when they reach the pinnacle of success, simply because their child-like features are flawless! Their skin is young, fresh and wrinkle-free. Modeling agencies use these perfect complexions like a painter uses a canvas. With makeup, hair and high-fashion clothing, agencies give these children an older or more sophisticated look. Keep this in mind when you are wondering what kind of attraction children can hold for even the biggest modeling agencies.

Plus-size Models —Who is a Candidate?

The physical characteristics of a plus-size model are the same as that of one in high-fashion, except they wear sizes 10-20. Your height should range from 5'9"-5'11"; you should weigh between 140-165; and you must be attractive. You should have long legs, which are proportionate to your body. Plus-size models are in demand more today than ever. Many of the top agencies in New York have added plus-size divisions. The types of work include catalog, ad campaigns and editorial. You are promoted just as high-fashion models are. And the advantage to being a plus-size model is that your age isn't as important as it is when trying to make it as a high-fashion model. There are successful, full-figured models who are over 40 years old. When you think about it, the majority of women over 40 are not pencil thin, and yet they have a desire to wear fashionable clothing.

Petite Models — Who is a Candidate?

Petite models range from 5'4" to 5'8". They are rarely seen on the catwalks in Paris, but are usually booked for beauty types of advertising. Their faces are seen on magazine covers, TV com-

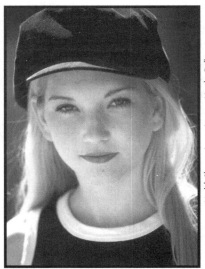
Model: Shauna Jones Agency: Marsha Doll
Agency Photographer: Mark Hanson

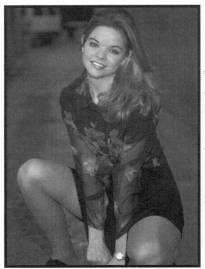
Model: Tamara Hardy Agency: Marsha Doll
Agency Photographer: Mark Hanson

mercials and product packaging. They're also marketed as young teens. Although most major designers offer petite lines, it's very tough to make it to super model status. But there is another area of the business where height is not a factor. TV commercials, soap operas and movies all use a wide range of looks. But to enter these markets, you better polish up on your acting skills.

Specialty Models — What Is Required?

Some people are recognized for having certain exceptional body parts, such as beautiful hands, legs, feet, eyes, lips, teeth or hair. Though being a specialty model requires real dedication to keep the specific body part in excellent physical condition, many models have turned specialty modeling into a real career! If you thrive on competition, being this type of model may be for you. As a specialty model, you will have to compete against the high-fashion models who are making their living promoting all parts of their bodies. Naturally, high-fashion models have several exceptionally beautiful body parts, and you may find it difficult to meet this challenge. There is always room in modeling for another candidate, however, and the pay for such an assignment is also exceptional! You will find that your salary for this type of job will often equal the pay that a fashion model would receive.

Just remember to stay active by keeping your asset(s) in the best condition possible. Pamper your legs, hands, eyes or whichever part you will use to earn your living. The hands you see in a dishwashing liquid commercial may one day be your own if you care for them well enough to hide any flaws from the camera! But, remember, even tiny scratches on your fingers can ruin your chances for an assignment. You will have to live in a large market place for this type of modeling to be a reality.

Male Modeling — Is There a Demand?

Now, more than ever, male models are making their mark in the modeling industry. Agents are looking for as many unique looks in men as they are in women. But there are still standards for male models, especially in high fashion. Most male models are 6'0" to 6'2" and wear between a size 40 - 42 coat. The most accepted pant size is 30" - 32" waist with a 32" - 34" inseam.

Model: Kevin Hannigan Agency: Marsha Doll Agency
Photographer: Mark Hanson

Did you notice anything peculiar about the size standards for male models? They're not required to be overly muscular. Though there are the Marky Marks and Tyson Beckfords in the modeling industry, most male models are lean and cut. You may think just because a guy is extremely muscular, he can be a model. The truth is, most male models are not muscular.

Model: Kobe Pigott Agency: Marsha Doll Agency Photographer: Mark Hanson

But if you don't fall into the high fashion standard, don't give up hope. The modeling industry offers you the same opportunities as it does to women. There is a market for big and tall men. There is print, television and film for men under the 6'0" standard (Tom Cruise is under 5'10"). And there is no limit or standard for character modeling.

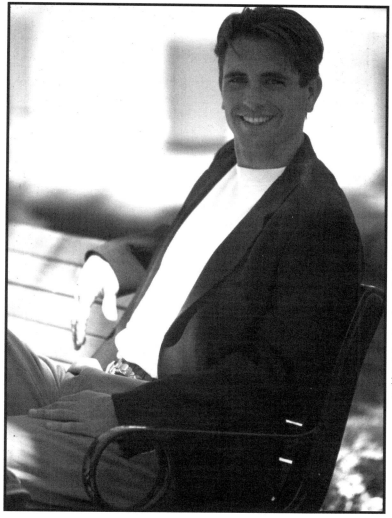

Model: Kevin Hannigan Agency: Marsha Doll Agency Photographer: Mark Hanson

Chapter 7
Making it as a Model

CHAPTER 7

MAKING IT AS A MODEL

Modeling Risks — Conventions, Searches, Photographers, etc.

In a profession like modeling, there exists incredible amounts of corruption. Because most people follow their hearts into such an uncertain lifestyle, they are willing to jump at any chance to become successful. The general public knows very little about modeling techniques and procedures, and some unscrupulous individuals are waiting to take advantage of this. It is in your best interest to be patient and to exercise extreme caution when dealing with people or circumstances with which you are unfamiliar.

My advice to you: Don't trust anyone until you are sure of his motives! Once you have been in the modeling business for a while, you will have the experience to make the right choices. Until then, play it safe and follow the conservative suggestions in this book and your own good, common sense.

First of all, stay away from newspaper ads reading, "Models Wanted." Professional and legitimate clients needing models will contact agencies to find them. Answering newspaper ads, in most cases, will not get you the type of modeling job you're looking for. As mentioned before, focus on the reputable agencies when you are first getting started so you don't get sidetracked into something that may turn out to be worthless or potentially dangerous.

Also, beware of so-called "model searches." There are so many traveling sideshows (model searches) these days. Many people are cashing in on these hotel types of conventions. They travel from city to city and hold these "big" interviews. Let's say 500 people attend, and they select 100 prospective models. They weed out people, making the ones who are chosen feel special. Once "selected," you will be expected to pay anywhere from $250 to

$500 to attend their convention. At the convention, large agency representatives will be present to "discover" new models. How could you possibly decline this opportunity? Though the big high-fashion agents will be there, the majority of the people "selected" to attend will never be high-fashion models. I have personally worked with many of these agents who have told me that they <u>do</u> find models they're interested in signing with their agency, but the percentage is small — very, very small. In fact, agents view these conventions as merely an opportunity to get out of the hustle-bustle of their everyday, hectic schedules with the hopes of finding that special new face.

Please remember, anyone who wants money up front for pictures, composites, promotion on the internet, training or any other promotional tool should be avoided. If the big agencies are sincerely interested in you, they will help you with your first set of pictures or charge a reasonable fee for testing. They believe in you and think you will make money. They will deduct the money they've invested in you from future earnings.

If you are truly interested in becoming a professional in this business, simply mail in snapshots. Another great way of being discovered is to enter contests which are legitimate and cost you absolutely nothing. Some of these reputable contests are sponsored by the "big" agencies in New York, such as Ford, Elite, Next and Wilhelmina.

There are people who can help you achieve your goals who will not require a "finder's fee" or some ridiculous amount of money. Small agencies, acting as scouts for larger agencies, receive a five percent commission from the agency, not the model. This is a great way for someone in a small or medium size market to break into the business on a larger scale.

Once you have become a professional model, you will have to pay your agent to represent you — this is expected at this point in your career and will be specified in your agency contract. An agency will not represent you without receiving a percentage (usually 20 to 25 percent) of your gross earnings. They are in the business of promoting you. How will you know the difference between a legitimate agency and a scam? You will. You will be able to make a wise decision based on what you have already learned about agencies through your experiences in the modeling world and this book.

Another mistake that unwary models often make is to give their telephone numbers and addresses out to anyone who asks for them. This is not a professional or a safe practice. If you meet someone new and are thinking about working with them, have your agency check his or her credentials. Or, if you have not yet signed with an agency, you may want to check with the Better Business Bureau or an equally reliable source. Please do this before providing anyone you don't know with any of your personal information.

What Can I Expect?

What can you expect to happen after you sign with an agency and are asked to come to a big city to work? Let's say you're with a successful school or small agency right now, and you're planning to send snapshots or visit a bigger agency where you hope to become recognized. If a scout likes your look, he or she may ask you to come to New York, Miami or Atlanta to do some test photography. The agency will possibly cover some of your expenses, including your testing. Once the pictures are finished they will determine whether you have what it takes to work for them! Pretty exciting? It gets better.

Model: Michelle Harwood Agency: Marsha Doll Agency Photographer: Mark Hanson

If an agency decides to sign you, you may be asked to spend time in Europe for some valuable experience that will prepare you for modeling under more rigorous conditions. Because there are so many more fashion magazines in Europe than in the U.S., your chances are much greater to get editorial work. This will give you a better chance of getting exposure and building your book, which is important for a model upon returning to New York. It will also give you more experience with professionals in the modeling industry, such as hairstylists, photographers and makeup artists. Then you can return to New York with a book full of tear sheets that will impress your potential clients. Not every agency will send you to Europe, but most suggest that it's worth your time to get tear sheets from places like Milan or Paris.

Going to Europe can seem intimidating to some, but many agencies pair two younger models together for long trips away from home. You can make the best of any situation, and Europe will prepare you for the stiff competition you can expect in New York. You will gain fantastic experience and tear sheets. From there it's on to future successes with your agency.

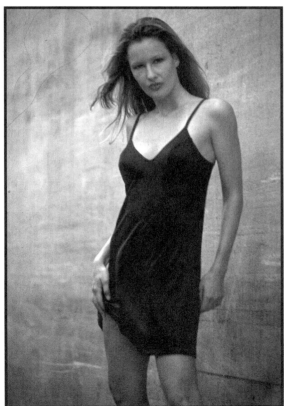

Model: Michelle Harwood Agency: Marsha Doll Agency
Photographer: Mark Hanson

Some hopeful models become sidetracked by what they consider to be a glamorous career full of parties, dates, business deals and the like. You may be tempted by all of this; however, you have to exercise some restraint. The most successful models are usually the ones who eat a healthy diet, take care of their bodies and generally get enough sleep to function properly.

Some models may be approached by big business clients or agency representatives who offer to help them find jobs in return for "personal favors." You do not have to resort to sex, drugs or other such behavior in order to become successful. That is not the way to become a model! Don't let anyone convince you that you need to do favors for them. You don't want assistance from anyone who would take advantage of you. Just as in any other career or business, models can be exposed to drug use and other vices, but if you respect yourself and keep your morals intact by using good judgment, you can succeed at anything.

How Much Money Do Models Make?

Some models make $15,000 to $250,000 per year; others don't make half that much. Then there are the ones who make over $1 million per year. It all depends on your look, your agency and where you're modeling. If you are lucky enough to be signed by an agency in New York, you can expect to make an average of $200 to $400 per day for editorial and $1,500 to $2,500 for catalog. As far as national television commercials go, you can make tens of thousands of dollars from the residuals alone. Residuals are the money you make every time your commercial is aired. Not bad money, is it?

Knowing the market, what lies ahead and how to get there is your first step. The rest is up to you. And please remember to stay focused, have a great attitude and be professional.

Chapter 8
Significant
Modeling Markets

SIGNIFICANT MODELING MARKETS

New York, New York

New York City is currently, and probably always will be, the center of activity for models. Because it is the primary location for aspiring and professional artists, photographers, musicians, actors, actresses and other hopeful "stars," everyone goes to New York to get the most exposure to the best opportunities. New York has so much potential. You may find that the rest of the nation looks to New York for the latest ideas and the greatest new fads. It's the cultural capital of the United States. If you become a 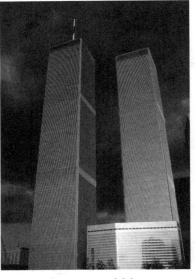 model in New York, you will have achieved an incredible accomplishment. The city is full of agencies, photographers, prospective clients and fashion designers. Because it houses all of these things on which models thrive, New York is every model's dream -- that's your ultimate destination.

New York is full of glamour, excitement, bright lights, eccentric people and large parties -- things that you might expect (sometimes incorrectly) from a life of modeling. The reality is, that while models may enjoy these things, usually their time is spent staying in shape to keep up with the increasing competition. In a situation where everyone flocks to the same location to try to achieve success, you must expect that the competition will be incredibly intense.

Even models from other big U.S. cities have trouble adjusting to life in New York. Everywhere you turn, another model is rising to popularity, landing a job that could have been yours! Even though modeling in New York is everyone's primary goal, it will not always be pleasant and productive. While it is the modeling center of the world, it can be a stressful place to live. If you enjoy a fast-paced way of life, New York may be just right for you.

Other Exciting Markets

Because New York's rigid standards are requiring more agencies and schools around the United States to improve their standards and to expect more from each model, other cities are rapidly expanding and becoming real alternatives in the modeling world. These cities include Miami, Atlanta, Dallas, Chicago, Los Angeles (primarily for film and television), Boston, Denver, Phoenix and Orlando. While they don't have the cultural flash that New York has to offer, these cities are certainly viable locations for upcoming, professional models.

Miami has become one of the hottest spots in the nation for modeling. Because of its beautiful, year-round climate, models can be photographed quickly and easily, saving the photographers (and everyone else involved) time and money. The European catalogs often shoot in Miami, as do many of the European magazines. Many models can get the experience they would have gained in Europe from the European clients who come to Miami. The models may be lucky enough to acquire a wide variety of tear sheets, since the European magazines and catalogs are produced so often. Models can really benefit from this type of opportunity!

If you are not from a large city, you may want to travel to one of these markets which is closest to your home. If this isn't an option, then get as much local and regional experience as possible. Again, check the list in the back of this book.

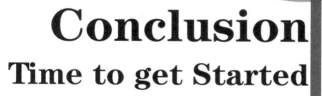

Conclusion
Time to get Started

TIME TO GET STARTED...

Now that you've read my basic advice for aspiring models, it's time for you to put this knowledge into action! Modeling is a real challenge, but it can be done if you've got the right attitude and are prepared for the business. Your own instincts will be your best guide when it comes to judging someone's character or deciding what school or agency is best for you.

It is my wish that this book has offered you a true understanding of the modeling world. You now have enough knowledge to make well-informed decisions. It is very important that you remember to get exposure when you are first starting out. The more exposure you get, the better your chances of becoming a model. I suggest you try one or more of the following:
1) Go through a smaller, reputable agency that has connections;
2) Send snapshots to agencies;
3) Enter the more prestigious contests sponsored by the big agencies and magazines; and/or
4) Go directly to New York (or another large market).
Traveling to a big city, as I've mentioned in earlier chapters, is going to cost more money since you will need to pay for travel and other expenses. Don't spend money on pictures — if a New York agency likes your appearance, they will do their own test shots, and your personal set of pictures won't be used at all. Use the list I've provided to help formulate a plan to become a model. The facts are all in front of you now, so put them to use. Remember, if it's character modeling you're interested in, all you need is a good black and white head shot and resume' to send to the various talent agencies.

As for modeling conventions associated with model searches, I suggest you stay away from them. Usually when you attend one of these conventions, your only opportunity to perform is when you walk out on stage holding a picture of yourself. There is another type of convention that you can attend only by way of your involvement with a reputable school/agency. These conventions are actually competitions and give out awards just like gymnastics, dance and other competitive activities. They are especially beneficial for people who are shy and unsure of themselves. The preparation necessary to perform at such a convention will do wonders for your self confidence. A good school or agency director will spend many hours working on such areas as your individual runway routine and television commercial. Just the experience of getting on stage in front of hundreds of people, including agents from all over the world, can be a major confidence builder for all ages. Don't go to any modeling convention with the hopes of becoming famous overnight.

In this book, I have stressed the importance of being cautious and persistent. If you can't attend a school or you can't travel, send your pictures to different agencies and follow up with telephone calls. Find out what is happening and what they think of you. Even if the answer isn't what you'd like to hear, you should not give up — the trends change every day, and tomorrow may be the day that a particular agency wants you to interview or sign with them! If you're rejected by the agencies, wait six months and try again.

If you're ever going to make it in the world of modeling, you can't give up on yourself. Modeling is a very tough business. I'm not being pessimistic, I'm being honest when I say very few people make a lifetime career of modeling. But always remember, with anything you try to achieve in life, don't let the rejection get to you. So many people expect good things to happen without putting forth any effort. Some of the most successful people in the world failed many times before they succeeded. You have to really like yourself and never give up. No one is going to knock on your door and say, "Hey! You're exactly who we've been looking for!" You have to go out there and make a difference. A good personality, the right attitude, an enormous amount of self confidence and the desire to achieve are essential.

Follow your dreams and never give up,

Marsha Doll-Faulkenberry

Modeling
Terms

MODELING TERMS

ADVERTISING LAYOUT - Production of an advertisement through art design.

AFTRA - American Federation of Television and Radio Artists — a union for various film and radio talent (see Chapter 5).

AGENT - A person or company that acts as a liaison for a model or an actor and assists them in obtaining job assignments. They usually earn a percentage of a model's salary, as specified by contract.

ART DIRECTOR - A person who handles creative artwork for an assignment.

BOOKINGS - A trade term meaning "job assignments."

"BREAK-IT-UP" - An expression used by photographers to mean "relax" while a model is working.

BUYER - An individual who purchases goods for a retail store, usually in bulk quantities.

CALL BACK - A second interview for a model.

CANCELLATION - A model's assignment is canceled after booking, due to complications.

CASTING DIRECTOR - A person who selects talent for film or modeling assignments.

CATALOG PHOTOGRAPHY - A photography shoot during which a model poses in an outfit to emphasize the garment's best qualities for use in a catalog.

CATTLE CALL - An audition for one job assignment which several models will attend.

COLLECTION (LINE) - A designer's group of fashions is his/her "collection." Moderately-priced clothing from one designer is called a "line."

COMMERCIAL ARTIST - A person who does advertising illustrations for magazines and other ad media.

COMMERCIAL MODEL - Special type of model needed for a specific assignment. Depending on the job description, this model could possess various characteristics and qualities — They may even be unattractive.

COMPOSITE - A model's "business card" — an 8" x 6" card containing his or her vital statistics and pictures for distribution to agencies and photographers (see Chapter 4).

CONTACT SHEET - Single 8" x 10" sheet of negative-produced proof photographs. A model can enlarge these proofs for use, if desired.

DESIGNER'S MODEL - A model who works exclusively for a designer to show collections to potential buyers.

EDITORIAL PHOTOGRAPHY (PRINT WORK) - Action posing for fashion assignments, not for advertisements. Crucial for building a good book.

EXHIBIT MODEL (CONVENTION MODEL) - Models/hosts or hostesses who work for conventions/promotions to hand out brochures and samples and to interact with customers in order to sell a particular product.

FASHION PHOTOGRAPHER - Takes photographs of a model for newspapers, retail store advertisements or magazines.

FASHION SHOW SEASONS (RETAIL) - Seasons when new fashions are shown. Holiday cruisewear fashions, November through January; spring & summer fashions, February through June; back to school and fall & winter fashions, August through November.

FASHION SHOW MODEL - Models who demonstrate new fashions before a live audience (see Chapter 5).

FASHION PHOTOGRAPHY MODEL - A model who poses for photography that may be displayed in newspapers, in retail advertisements, or in catalogs, for example.

FITTING MODEL - A model who allows designers to use his or her body for fitting of new fashions. He or she stands while the designer creates fashion on her/him.

FREELANCE MODEL - A model who either works with several agencies at once or who is independent and searches for his or her own assignments, free of contract restrictions (see Chapter 1).

"GO SEE" - A trade term meaning to interview for a possible assignment.

HIGH-FASHION MODEL - A model who satisfies certain physical criteria for being tall, sophisticated and dramatic (see Chapter 2).

INDUSTRIAL FILMS - Educational movies or slides that privately promote a company's products or services.

ILLUSTRATIVE MODEL - A model who poses with a product — not usually in a high-fashion capacity.

INTERVIEW ("GO SEE") - A job assignment audition.

JUNIOR MODEL - A young-looking, teenage model. Usually small boned, 5'4" - 5'6", and wears clothing sizes 3, 5 or 7. Age usually ranges from 15 - 18.

JUNIOR PETITE MODEL - A model who must be under 5'4" for fashion work and usually wears sizes 3, 5 or 7.

MAKEUP ARTIST - An expert who applies makeup for modeling assignments (usually they are freelance).

MISSES MODEL - A model who is older looking, taller than a junior model and wears misses sizes 8, 10, 12 or 14.

MODEL AGENCY - A professional company designed to register, promote, hire and pay different types of models. They usually receive a portion of a model's earnings, as specified by contract (see Chapter 1).

MATRON MODEL (MOTHER-OF-THE-BRIDE MODEL) - A mature, attractive model who is able to wear misses/larger sizes (14 - 16)) or half sizes (14 1/2 - 16 1/2).

PRESS SHOWING - Showings of upcoming fashions for members of the press.

PROOFS - (see Contact sheets).

PORTFOLIO (BOOK) - A book of plastic inserts containing pictures of a model. Always take your portfolio to interviews.

PRE-TEEN MODEL - A model who must appear to be between the ages of 9-12. This type of model typically does fashion, photographic and commercial work.

RETAIL MODELING (FASHION) - A model who demonstrates clothing provided by a dress salon or a department store.

RESIDUALS - Money that a radio or television model receives every time his or her particular advertisement is played.

RESUME' (MODELING) - Information sheet giving the complete history, statistics and assignments done by a model.

s.f. - Small-lettered abbreviation for "stocking feet." Relates to the height of the model.

SAMPLE MODEL - A model on whom a designer's original sample dress was made.

SPECIALTY MODEL - A model who capitalizes on some very exceptional body parts — feet, hair, eyes, hands, etc. (see Chapter 6).

STYLIST - With a sharp eye for details, he/she makes certain the movie or photography set is perfect.

TEA ROOM (INFORMAL) MODEL - A model who models clothes informally during special events, luncheons or dinners. Interacts with prospective buyers.

TEAR SHEETS - Photos a model keeps of himself/herself that have appeared in print media.

TV COMMERCIALS - Models talk and/or act to sell a product on TV.

TEST SHOTS - Pictures that photographers take of models to test ideas.

TINY-TOT MODEL - A model who must appear to be 4 - 8 years old. He or she typically does fashion, commercial or photographic work.

TRUNK SHOWING - A designer's original collection, shipped (in a trunk) to various cities to be shown to prospective buyers.

SCREENING - Interviewing many models and selecting most suitable for the job.

VOICE OVER - A model's voice being used for another model being filmed or photographed for a commercial.

VOUCHER - A three-copy receipt a model receives from an agency to have signed at the end of an assignment. Client and model both sign an agreement of hours and fees.

WHOLESALE MODEL - A model who works for a manufacturer in the wholesale salon (apparel centers or marts) where buyers place orders.

FILM TERMS

AGENT - Person(s) responsible for arranging actors' auditions and maintaining their careers.

AUDIO - The sound portion of a radio or television production.

AUDITION - A scheduled opportunity for testing an actor's talent.

B.G. - BACKGROUND - Sound used as a background effect (could also refer to the presence of "extras" on the set).

BIT - A small part in the production of a movie.

CAMERA LEFT - Movement to your right (when facing camera) - same as stage left.

CAMERA RIGHT - Movement to your left (when facing camera) - same as stage right.

CAMERA REHEARSAL - A complete rehearsal with cameras and actors, usually a dress rehearsal.

CASTING - Choosing a specific model to represent a stereotype or character in a film production — usually done by the casting director.

CASTING DIRECTOR - Person(s) who chooses actors for film roles.

CHALK - Used to mark performers' correct position in front of the cameras and on the stage.

CHARACTER - A person who appears in a script and is often defined by a particular stereotype or a certain image. They are usually recognized by specific physiological or emotional traits.

CHEAT - Angling an actor or an object toward a certain camera without the knowledge of the audience.

CLAP STICK(S) - Device that helps with the development of sound in a film production — (You may remember this object as a black and white slate that claps together during "take one," for example.)

CLIENT - A person or an agency interested in hiring actors and actresses to represent a particular idea or product.

COMMENTARY - A description of clothing worn in a fashion show, typically read by the commentator.

COMMISSION - A percentage of actors' fees that is required to be paid to an agency, as specified by contract.

CONTROL ROOM - A room filled with production technology and equipment that is in view of the actors. The film production crew uses this room as a place to perform their production duties.

CREDITS - Job assignments which an actor has completed and for which he or she has been paid.

CREW - Personnel involved in the production of a film.

CROSS OVER (X) - An actor's movement across a stage.

CUE - The beginning of the film action.

CUT - A signal by the director to end the action of a film.

DISSOLVE - The slow and simultaneous replacement of one film scene with a concurrent scene.

DOLLY SHOT - A scene in which the camera is mounted on a moving tripod, facilitating easy movement of the camera either closer to or further from the source of the action.

DOWN STAGE - Position nearest the front of the stage and the audience.

EXTRA - An actor's minor role in a film. Usually an actor is an "extra" in his or her first film experience.

FEES (RATES) - The amount of money an actor generates for his or her work.

FRAME - The area pictured within the camera lens.

HAND PROPS - Various objects that are held or demonstrated by the actor during a film or a commercial.

"IT'S A WRAP" - A verbal sign from the director that the day's work (or the entire film project) is over.

LINE - Dialogue spoken by an actor.

LOCATION - Place at which a movie or a commercial is being filmed.

MARK - Chalk or tape mark that indicates where an actor should stand.

RELEASE - A contract signed by an actor that allows his or her work to be released to others, as the client specifies.

MOOD - A feeling that an actor must project to the audience.

OFF CAMERA - Performance that is purposely not included on camera, like narration, for example.

OPEN CALL - Casting which all may attend.

PAN SHOT - The camera moves in certain directions (right or left) to follow an action that is taking place.

PICKUP - Beginning the action again from a point at which an error was made.

PRINCIPAL ROLE - The main movie role.

"PRINT IT" - A cue from a director to save a particular piece of film for future use.

PRODUCTION COMPANY - A company responsible for the technical aspects of film or movie production.

PROJECT - Enunciation or expression of feelings or attitudes by an actor.

QUICK STUDY - An actor capable of memorizing complex lines; one who has an aptitude for acting.

RISER PLATFORM - A platform used to bring actors to a specific height.

ROUNDS - Approaching prospective clients for work ("making the rounds").

RUN-THROUGH - An actor's rehearsal.

SET - The situation of scenery to make an impression on the audience; the place where the action is performed.

SHOT - Trade term for "a picture."

SLATE - The bottom portion of a clapstick that lists the scene numbers and other pertinent information for the actors and directors.

S.O.F. - Sound on film.

S.O.T. - Sound on tape.

STAGE OR STUDIO DIRECTIONS - Directions given to an actor to inform him or her where to move on the set (see STAGE LEFT/STAGE RIGHT).

STAND-BY - A cue, usually verbal, that action is about to take place.

STAND-IN - A person who replaces an actor for tedious film work.

STRIKE IT - A cue from the director to remove or delete a certain portion from the film.

TAKE - A scene in which the action can be photographed many times, and only the best "take" will be used in the film or in the commercial.

TALENT - A term that often means "performers."

TELEPROMPTER - A screen similar to a TV set from which actors read their lines.

TRACK - A portion of video or film which carries the sound.

TYPECASTING - Placing an actor in a role for which he or she is perfectly matched by his or her everyday actions and feelings.

UPSTAGE - Movement toward the back of the set and away from the audience.

VOICE OVER (V.0. or V/0) - Off-screen narration.

ZOOM SHOT - A special lens shot in which an object moves either toward or away from the camera. Though it is similar, it is not the same as a DOLLY SHOT.

Directory

Directory

For your convenience, I have indicated with an * (asterisk) the agencies my company is familiar with. Once again, I do not necessarily recommend these agencies. Use your own good judgment and discretion.

ALASKA

ALASKA MODELS & TALENT 601 W 41ST AVE # 204 ANCHORAGE AK 99503 (907) 561-5739

JOHN ROBERT POWERS MODELING 300 E DIMOND BLVD ANCHORAGE AK 99515 (907) 344-2525

MODEL PERFECT THE AGENCY PO Box 211311 ANCHORAGE AK 99515 (917) 258-7600

NORTHERN STARS PO BOX 770369 EAGLE RIVER AK 99577 (907) 688-1370

ARIA STUDIOS 2120 S CUSHMAN ST # 210 FAIRBANKS AK 99701 (907) 456-8959

ALABAMA

ACADEMY OF FINE ARTS 2026 2ND AVE N BIRMINGHAM AL 35203 (205) 320-0888

ATLANTA TALENT CONSULTANTS 5813 53RD AVE N BIRMINGHAM AL 35217 (205) 849-9806

CATHI LARSEN AGENCY 1628 6th St. N.W. BIRMINGHAM AL 35215 (205) 951-2445

ELAN AGENCY 1446 Montgomery Hwy BIRMINGHAM AL 35216 (205) 823-9180

INTERNATIONAL IMAGE MODEL AGCY 616 RED LANE RD BIRMINGHAM AL 35215 (205) 836-1030

KIDDIN' AROUND MODELS & TALENT 700 S 28TH ST # 210 BIRMINGHAM AL 35233 (205) 323-5437

MODELS & MODELS 1920 OXMOOR RD BIRMINGHAM AL 35209 (205) 879-3441

PLANET MODEL & TALENT MGMT 6 55TH PL S BIRMINGHAM AL 35212 (205) 592-6542

STAR QUALITY TALENT AGENCY 1316 STRATFORD RD SE DECATUR AL 35601 (205) 350-6005

RARE QUALITY MODELS & TALENT 260 N. Foster St. DOTHAN AL 36303 (334) 671-2200

CHRIS & CO 5500 MYRON MASSEY BLVD FAIRFIELD AL 35064 (205) 780-0032

IMAGE MAKERS INC 7500 MEMORIAL PKY SW HUNTSVILLE AL 35802 (205) 880-9050

PAMA STUDIO 721 CLINTON AVE W HUNTSVILLE AL 35801 (205) 536-5200

PAZAZZ MODELS-TALENT TRAINING 4367 DOWNTOWNER LOOP N MOBILE AL 36609 (334) 343-2502

TALENT SOUTH MODELING 3350 COTTAGE HILL RD MOBILE AL 36606 (334) 476-0420

ALABAMA-ATLANTA CASTING SVC 380 MENDEL PKY W MONTGOMERY AL 36117 (334) 244-4464

CYNTHIA'S STUDIO 2030 E 4TH ST MONTGOMERY AL 36106 (334) 272-5555

RARE QUALITY MODELS & TALENT 380 MENDEL PKY W MONTGOMERY AL 36117 (334) 244-4464

READY FOR THE WORLD MODELING 4429 TROY HWY MONTGOMERY AL 36116 (334) 284-3006

STAR TREE TALENT 173 W MAIN ST PRATTVILLE AL 36067 (334) 361-6363

ALABAMA TALENT MANAGEMENT 621 22ND AVE TUSCALOOSA AL 35401 (205) 364-8700

Arkansas

MODEL 1 1202 N HIGHLAND AVE EL DORADO AR 71730 (501) 862-1914

BROOKS MODELING AGENCY 320 OUACHITA AVE # 315 HOT SPRINGS AR 71901 (501) 321-0202

CROWN AGENCY 309 WHITTINGTON AVE HOT SPRINGS AR 71901 (501) 623-5911

RON BEEMAN MODELING AGENCY 1306 GOLF LINKS RD HOT SPRINGS AR 71901 (501) 624-6988

AGENCY INC 910 W 6TH ST LITTLE ROCK AR 72201 (501) 374-6447

BELLES & BEAUS MODELING TROUPE 8703 KANIS RD LITTLE ROCK AR 72204 (501) 221-9131

FERGUSON MODELING & TALENT 1100 W 34TH ST LITTLE ROCK AR 72206 (501) 375-3519

TERRY LONG MODELS PO BOX 7353 LITTLE ROCK AR 72217 (501) 221-2202

Arizona

DANI'S AGENCY 1 E CAMELBACK RD # 550 PHOENIX AZ 85012 (602) 263-1918

INTERNATIONAL TALENT MGMT PO BOX 9250 PHOENIX AZ 85068 (602) 943-2700

JEAN FOWLER COACH WORKS 3033 N 44TH ST PHOENIX AZ 85018 (602) 952-8493

*LEIGHTON AGENCY INC 2231 E. Camelback Rd. #319 PHOENIX AZ 85016 (602) 224-9255

MODELS FOR HIRE PROMOTIONAL 1555 E GLENDALE AVE PHOENIX AZ 85020 (602) 994-0880

REEL PEOPLE 5031 N 34TH ST PHOENIX AZ 85018 (602) 994-9300

SIGNATURE MODELS & TALENT AGCY 2600 N 44TH ST # 209 PHOENIX AZ 85008 (602) 966-1102

TOR-ANN TALENT & BOOKING AGNCY 6711 N 21ST WAY PHOENIX AZ 85016 (602) 263-8708

VOICE CASTING HOUSE 1236 E NORTHERN AVE # 2 PHOENIX AZ 85020 (602) 371-0139

PINE MOUNTAIN TALENT 1042 WILLOW CREEK RD # 1-301 PRESCOTT AZ 86301 (520) 771-1380

ARIZONA MEDIA RESOURCES 7373 E SCOTTSDALE MALL SCOTTSDALE AZ 85251 (602) 994-1255

COSMOS MODEL & TALENT 4141 N GOLDWATER BLVD # 101 SCOTTSDALE AZ 85251 (602) 949-6004

ELIZABETH SAVAGE TALENT AGENCY 4949 E LINCOLN DR SCOTTSDALE AZ 85253 (602) 840-3530

J & J INTL MODEL & TALENT 7120 E 6TH AVE SCOTTSDALE AZ 85251 (602) 945-1005

MODEL & TALENT MANAGEMENT 4533 N SCOTTSDALE RD # 201 SCOTTSDALE AZ 85251 (602) 941-4941

NETWORK INTERNATIONAL MODELS 4300 N MILLER RD # 242 SCOTTSDALE AZ 85251 (602) 941-6922

*ROBERT FORD BLACK AGENCY 7525 E CAMELBACK RD # 200 SCOTTSDALE AZ 85251 (602) 966-2537

STARMAKER MODELS & TALENT 4223 N SCOTTSDALE RD SCOTTSDALE AZ 85251 (602) 949-0180

AVOLIO INTERNATIONAL 944 S MILL AVE TEMPE AZ 85281 (602) 784-5900

MODEL SEARCH MAGAZINE 822 S MILL AVE # 115 TEMPE AZ 85281 (602) 897-2887

ACT THEATRICAL & MODELING 6264 E GRANT RD TUCSON AZ 85712 (520) 885-3246

ACTOR'S AGENCY 2910 N SWAN RD # 110 TUCSON AZ 85712 (520) 321-1973

BARAKA TALENT AGENCY 3210 E FORT LOWELL RD TUCSON AZ 85716 (520) 795-1909

FLAIR PARISIENNE DRAMA STUDIOS 6700 N ORACLE RD # 501 TUCSON AZ 85704 (520) 742-1090

FOSI'S TALENT AGENCY 2777 N CAMPBELL AVE TUCSON AZ 85719 (520) 795-3534

MEDJURAN MODELING & TALENT 1790 E RIVER RD TUCSON AZ 85718 (520) 577-5143

TOM THUMB PLAYERS CO 6264 E GRANT RD TUCSON AZ 85712 (520) 885-3246

California

SYD LEWIS TALENT AGENCY PO BOX 970 ANAHEIM CA 92815 (714) 971-5004

STUDIO TEACHER 120 LINDA CT APTOS CA 95003 (408) 685-1410

EXTRAORDINAIRE MODELS 200 NEW STINE RD BAKERSFIELD CA 93309 (805) 397-4440

MC CRIGHT MODELING SCHOOL 1011 STINE RD BAKERSFIELD CA 93309 (805) 835-1305

ALLEN BONNI TALENT AGENCY 260 S BEVERLY DR BEVERLY HILLS CA 90212 (310) 247-1865

AMBROSIO-MORTIMER & ASSOC 9150 WILSHIRE BLVD # 175 BEVERLY HILLS CA 90212 (310) 274-4274

BARRY SECUNDA ASSOC 321 S BEVERLY DR BEVERLY HILLS CA 90212 (310) 785-0444

BELSON & KLASS ASSOC 144 S BEVERLY DR # 405 BEVERLY HILLS CA 90212 (310) 274-9169

BETH CANNON CO 250 N ROBERTSON BLVD BEVERLY HILLS CA 90211 (310) 276-6144

BLAKE AGENCY 415 N CAMDEN DR BEVERLY HILLS CA 90210 (310) 246-0241

BLOOM AT FORD 88826 BURTON WAY BEVERLY HILLS CA 90011 (310) 276-8100

CIRCLE TALENT ASSOC 433 N CAMDEN DR BEVERLY HILLS CA 90210 (310) 285-1585

COLOR ME BRIGHT TALENT AGENCY 433 N CAMDEN DR BEVERLY HILLS CA 90210 (310) 858-1681

COMMERCIALS UNLIMITED 9601 WILSHIRE BLVD BEVERLY HILLS CA 90210 (310) 888-8788

CREATIVE CHILDREN'S MANAGEMENT 345 S ELM DR BEVERLY HILLS CA 90212 (310) 859-7100

DEE'S KIDS & SENIOR CITIZEN 8693 WILSHIRE BLVD BEVERLY HILLS CA 90211 (310) 652-4695

DOROTHY DAY OTIS & ASSOC 373 S ROBERTSON BLVD BEVERLY HILLS CA 90211 (818) 905-9510

DOUGLAS AGENCY 211 S BEVERLY DR BEVERLY HILLS CA 90212 (310) 888-8822

ELITE MODEL MANAGEMENT 345 N MAPLE DR BEVERLY HILLS CA 90210 (310) 274-9395

*ELITE NEW FACES 345 N MAPLE DR # 397 BEVERLY HILLS CA 90210 (310) 859-7767

*FORD MODELS, INC. 88826 BURTON WAY BEVERLY HILLS CA 90211 (310) 276-8100

GELLER MEDIA MANAGEMENT INC 9454 WILSHIRE BLVD # 600 BEVERLY HILLS CA 90212 (310) 271-7900

GERSH AGENCY INC 232 N CANON DR BEVERLY HILLS CA 90210 (310) 274-6611

*GILLA ROOS WEST 9744 WILSHIRE BLVD #203 BEVERLY HILLS CA 90212 (310) 274-9356

GLAMOUR MODELS CASTING 211 S BEVERLY DR # 110 BEVERLY HILLS CA 90212 (310) 859-4899

HELLER SEYMOUR N 520 N CAMDEN DR BEVERLY HILLS CA 90210 (310) 271-8087

HOWARD ROSE AGENCY LTD 8900 WILSHIRE BLVD # 320 BEVERLY HILLS CA 90211 (310) 657-1215

INTERNATIONAL CREATIVE MGMT 8942 WILSHIRE BLVD BEVERLY HILLS CA 90211 (310) 550-4000

IRV SCHECHTER CO 9300 WILSHIRE BLVD # 400 BEVERLY HILLS CA 90212 (310) 278-8070

IRVIN ARTHUR ASSOC 9363 WILSHIRE BLVD BEVERLY HILLS CA 90210 (310) 278-5934

LARRY LARSON & ASSOC PO BOX 10905 BEVERLY HILLS CA 90213 (310) 271-7240

LEWIS & QUINN 9812 W OLYMPIC BLVD BEVERLY HILLS CA 90212 (310) 552-9412

LOU ALEXANDER AGENCY 211 S BEVERLY DR BEVERLY HILLS CA 90212 (310) 859-8701

LW1 TALENT 8383 WILSHIRE BLVD # 649 BEVERLY HILLS CA 90211 (213) 653-5700

MAC MODELING 9454 WILSHIRE BLVD # 720 BEVERLY HILLS CA 90212 (310) 273-2566

MADEMOISELLE MODELING AGENCY 8693 WILSHIRE BLVD BEVERLY HILLS CA 90211 (310) 289-8005

MAJOR CLIENTS AGENCY 345 N MAPLE DR BEVERLY HILLS CA 90210 (310) 205-5000

MARTIN MANAGEMENTS 9100 WILSHIRE BLVD # 401E BEVERLY HILLS CA 90212 (310) 247-0934

MEINIKER MANAGEMENT 209 S RODEO DR BEVERLY HILLS CA 90212 (310) 553-0987

MERIDIAN TALENT AGENCY 499 N. CANON DRIVE BEVERLY HILLS CA 90210 (310) 652-7799

MICHAEL NORTH CO 315 S BEVERLY DR # 206 BEVERLY HILLS CA 90212 (310) 277-9124

MICHELLE GORDON & ASSOC 260 S BEVERLY DR # 308 BEVERLY HILLS CA 90212 (310) 246-9930

OUTPOST MANAGEMENT 8601 WILSHIRE BLVD BEVERLY HILLS CA 90211 (310) 289-8004

PRITCHER CO 409 N CAMDEN DR BEVERLY HILLS CA 90210 (310) 247-8088

PROGRESSIVE ARTISTS 400 S BEVERLY DR # 216 BEVERLY HILLS CA 90212 (310) 553-8561

ROBIN LEVY & ASSOC INC 9701 WILSHIRE BLVD BEVERLY HILLS CA 90212 (310) 278-8748

RON RAINEY MANAGEMENT 315 S BEVERLY DR # 206 BEVERLY HILLS CA 90212 (310) 557-0661

ROTHMAN AGENCY 9401 WILSHIRE BLVD # 830 BEVERLY HILLS CA 90212 (310) 247-9898

SARKES KERNIS SECUNDA 321 S BEVERLY DR BEVERLY HILLS CA 90212 (310) 785-0444

SCREEN ARTISTS TALENT 8907 WILSHIRE BLVD BEVERLY HILLS CA 90211 (310) 358-7252

SHAPIRO-WEST & ASSOC INC 141 S EL CAMINO DR # 205 BEVERLY HILLS CA 90212 (310) 278-8896

SIRENS MODEL MANAGEMENT 9455 SANTA MONICA BLVD BEVERLY HILLS CA 90210 (310) 246-1969

SONJIA BRANDON'S 9601 WILSHIRE BLVD # 620 BEVERLY HILLS CA 90210 (310) 888-8788

STAN IRWIN ENTERPRISES INC 8484 WILSHIRE BLVD BEVERLY HILLS CA 90211 (213) 651-0315

SUSAN SMITH & ASSOC 121 N SAN VICENTE BLVD BEVERLY HILLS CA 90211 (213) 852-4777

TALENT GROUP INC 6300 WILSHIRE BLVD # 2110 BEVERLY HILLS CA 90212 (213) 852-9559

THOMAS-ROSSON AGENCY 124 S LASKY DR BEVERLY HILLS CA 90212 (310) 247-2727

UNITED TALENT 9560 WILSHIRE BLVD # 500 BEVERLY HILLS CA 90212 (310) 273-6700

US TALENT AGENCY 485 S. ROBERTSON, SUITE 7 BEVERLY HILLS CA 90211 (310) 858-7220

WAX AGENCY 120 S EL CAMINO DR # 114 BEVERLY HILLS CA 90212 (310) 550-8738

*WILHELMINA MODELS INC 8383 WILSHIRE BLVD # 650 BEVERLY HILLS CA 90211 (213) 655-0909

*WILLIAM MORRIS AGENCY INC 151 S EL CAMINO DR BEVERLY HILLS CA 90212 (310) 859-4000

WOMEN & MEN AT LARGE PO BOX 2572 BEVERLY HILLS CA 90213 (310) 278-9902

BONNIE BLACK TALENT AGENCY 4405 W RIVERSIDE DR BURBANK CA 91505 (818) 840-1299

CENEX CASTING 1700 W BURBANK BLVD BURBANK CA 91506 (818) 562-2800

CENTRAL CASTING 1700 W BURBANK BLVD BURBANK CA 91506 (818) 562-2700

COLLEEN CLER MODELING INST 120 S VICTORY BLVD BURBANK CA 91502 (818) 841-7943

GOLD-MARSHAK & ASSOC 3500 W OLIVE AVE BURBANK CA 91505 (818) 972-4300

GUY LEE & ASSOC 4150 W RIVERSIDE DR # 212 BURBANK CA 91505 (818) 848-7475

HOLLYWOOD STUDIOS PO BOX 285 BURBANK CA 91503 (818) 563-4289

JAMES LEVY JACOBSON 3500 W OLIVE AVE BURBANK CA 91505 (818) 955-7070

SCREEN CHILDREN'S AGENCY 4000 W RIVERSIDE DR BURBANK CA 91505 (818) 846-4300

SIPOLE LAYNE MANAGEMENT 4150 W RIVERSIDE DR # 208 BURBANK CA 91505 (818) 557-1570

WILLIAM CARROLL AGENCY 139 N SAN FERNANDO BLVD BURBANK CA 91502 (818) 845-3791

DON ANDERSON PRODUCTIONS INC 840 MALCOLM RD BURLINGAME CA 94010 (415) 692-9444

ED JESSWANI PRODUCTIONS 1290 BAYSHORE HWY BURLINGAME CA 94010 (415) 343-3851

ELLICOTT TALENT GROUP 2209 ADELINE DR BURLINGAME CA 94010 (415) 347-9624

SHANNON GREEN TALENT 205 PARK RD BURLINGAME CA 94010 (415) 348-2121

BEVERLY AGENCY 371 MOBIL AVE CAMARILLO CA 93010 (805) 445-9262

PROGRESSIVE MODELS 3615 LAS POSAS RD CAMARILLO CA 93010 (805) 484-5434

BARBARA CAMERON & ASSOC INC 8369 SAUSALITO AVE CANOGA PARK CA 91304 (818) 888-6107

ELEGANCE MODELING STUDIO 2763 STATE ST CARLSBAD CA 92008 (619) 434-3397

HANK RITTER MODEL MANAGEMENT 3528 WINSTON WAY CARMICHAEL CA 95608 (916) 487-1991

AKO PRODUCTIONS 20531 PLUMMER ST CHATSWORTH CA 91311 (818) 998-0443

MASTORAKIS ANDREAS 15696 ALTAMIRA DR CHINO CA 91709 (909) 597-3160

ONAC PRODUCTIONS 664 MARSAT CT CHULA VISTA CA 91911 (619) 575-7247

NATIONAL SCHOLARSHIP PAGEANT PO BOX 422 CITRUS HEIGHTS CA 95611 (916) 728-5824

KEVIN LYMAN PRODUCTION SVC 112 HARVARD AVE # 244 CLAREMONT CA 91711 (909) 626-4245

PEET-U TALENT AGENCY 831 W VALLEY BLVD COLTON CA 92324 (909) 783-2723

INTERNATN'L COVER MOD SRCH 19800 MACARTHUR BLVD # 500 COSTA MESA CA 92626 (714) 540-9203

MARIAN BERZON TALENT 336 E 17TH ST COSTA MESA CA 92627 (714) 631-5936

MORGAN AGENCY 129 W WILSON ST COSTA MESA CA 92627 (714) 574-1100

A TO Z TALENT 1051 N CITRUS AVE COVINA CA 91722 (818) 859-3335

PARK AVENUE IMAGES 557 N AZUSA AVE COVINA CA 91722 (818) 915-4957

DORIE TALENT AGENCY 11750 DUBLIN BLVD DUBLIN CA 94568 (510) 563-4747

WORLD CLASS SPORTS 880 APOLLO ST # 337 EL SEGUNDO CA 90245 (310) 278-2010

BRESLER KELLY & ASSOC 15760 VENTURA BLVD ENCINO CA 91436 (818) 905-1155

C C TALENT 16055 VENTURA BLVD ENCINO CA 91436 (818) 905-0102

HARRISON GROUP LTD 15720 VENTURA BLVD # 105 ENCINO CA 91436 (818) 379-9700

STARMAKER 15467 HAMPTON CT FONTANA CA 92337 (909) 428-9951

AMERICAN MISS PAGEANT SYSTEM 6046 N HAZEL AVE FRESNO CA 93711 (209) 436-1667

CENTRAL VALLEY CASTING 2002 N GATEWAY BLVD # 105 FRESNO CA 93727 (209) 455-0756

DE VORE ARTISTS TALENT 2236 N FINE AVE FRESNO CA 93727 (209) 255-2317

J M TALENT MANAGEMENT 4793 E SHIELDS AVE FRESNO CA 93726 (209) 452-0172

LITTLE MISS AMERICA 4141 E GETTYSBURG AVE FRESNO CA 93726 (209) 224-2883

REFLECTIONS MODELING 13971 VAN NESS AVE GARDENA CA 90249 (310) 329-2996

BERZON AGENCY 1614 VICTORY BLVD GLENDALE CA 91201 (818) 548-1560

BERZON TALENT AGENCY 1614 VICTORY BLVD GLENDALE CA 91201 (818) 552-2699

LEE S MIMMS & ASSOC INC 2644 E CHEVY CHASE DR GLENDALE CA 91206 (818) 246-5601

DSW FILM ACTORS WORKSHOP 509 E ALOSTA AVE GLENDORA CA 91740 (818) 963-3999

MEDIA CASTING 6963 DOUGLAS BLVD # 294 GRANITE BAY CA 95746 (916) 925-0196

DOUG MORRISSON THEATRICAL 22732 FOOTHILL BLVD HAYWARD CA 94541 (510) 886-9222

ACTOR'S STUDIO WEST 16582 GOTHARD ST HUNTINGTON BEACH CA 92647 (714) 969-2278

BRAND MODEL & TALENT AGENCY 17941 SKY PARK CIR IRVINE CA 92614 (714) 251-0555

EL TORO MODELS GUILD 15500 ROCKFIELD BLVD IRVINE CA 92618 (714) 837-9903

MISS & TEEN SOUTH ORANGE CO PO BOX 51583 IRVINE CA 92619 (714) 662-7696

PROFILE 204 W YALE LOOP IRVINE CA 92604 (714) 651-6050

TANNER MODELS 2102 BUSINESS CTR IRVINE CA 92612 (714) 253-5752

ACTION TALENT AGENCY 4342 OAKWOOD AVE LA CANADA CA 91011 (818) 790-4616

CES 7825 FAY AVE LA JOLLA CA 92037 (619) 456-5580

JET SET MANAGEMENT 7855 FAY AVE, #350 LA JOLLA CA 92038 (619) 551-9393

JANE DEACY AGENCY INC 4615 SKYLINE LN LA MESA CA 91941 (619) 698-6620

LET'S FACE IT 570 CENTRAL AVE LAKE ELSINORE CA 92530 (909) 245-6500

CHIC MODELING 236 QUINCY AVE LONG BEACH CA 90803 (310) 438-5088

ABRAMS-RUBALOFF & LAWRENCE INC 8075 W 3RD ST LOS ANGELES CA 90048 (213) 935-1700

AFH TALENT AGENCY 8240 BEVERLY BLVD LOS ANGELES CA 90048 (213) 932-6042

AGENCY FOR THE PERFORM ARTS 9000 W SUNSET BLVD # 1200 LOS ANGELES CA 90069 (310) 273-0744

ALLMAN MANAGEMENT 342 S COCHRAN AVE LOS ANGELES CA 90036 (213) 965-0967

ANALISE COLLINS CASTING 1103 N EL CENTRO AVE LOS ANGELES CA 90038 (213) 962-9562

ARLENE L DAYTON MANAGEMENT INC 10110 EMPYREAN WAY LOS ANGELES CA 90067 (310) 277-1266

ARLENE THORNTON & ASSOC 5657 WILSHIRE BLVD # 290 LOS ANGELES CA 90036 (213) 939-5757

ARMENIAN AMERICAN THEATRICAL 3111 LOS FELIZ BLVD LOS ANGELES CA 90039 (213) 668-1030

ARTIST NETWORK 8438 MELROSE PL LOS ANGELES CA 90069 (213) 651-4244

ARTISTS AGENCY 10000 SANTA MONICA BLVD # 305 LOS ANGELES CA 90067 (310) 277-7779

ARTISTS GROUP LTD 10100 SANTA MONICA BLVD # 2490 LOS ANGELES CA 90067 (310) 552-1100

ATKINS & ASSOC 303 S CRESCENT HEIGHTS BLVD LOS ANGELES CA 90048 (213) 658-1021

BAIER-KLEINMAN INTL 3575 CAHUENGA BLVD W LOS ANGELES CA 90068 (213) 874-4872

BALDWIN TALENT INC 500 S SEPULVEDA BLVD # 4 LOS ANGELES CA 90049 (310) 472-7919

BARBIZON SCHOOL OF MODELING 3450 WILSHIRE BLVD # 415 LOS ANGELES CA 90010 (213) 487-1500

BASS INTERNATIONAL MODEL SCOUT 10877 PALMS BLVD LOS ANGELES CA 90034 (310) 839-1097

BAUMAN HILLER & ASSOC 5757 WILSHIRE BLVD # 5 LOS ANGELES CA 90036 (213) 857-6666

BENSON AGENCY 8360 MELROSE AVE LOS ANGELES CA 90069 (213) 653-0500

BEVERLY HILLS MODEL & TALENT 8360 MELROSE AVE LOS ANGELES CA 90069 (213) 653-7655

BEVERLY LONG & ASSOC 6671 W SUNSET BLVD LOS ANGELES CA 90028 (213) 466-0770

BIL-MAR PRODUCTIONS 8929 S SEPULVEDA BLVD # 314 LOS ANGELES CA 90045 (310) 338-9602

BILL DANCE CASTING 3518 CAHUENGA BLVD W LOS ANGELES CA 90068 (213) 878-1131

BOPLA TALENT AGENCY 1467 TAMARIND AVE LOS ANGELES CA 90028 (213) 466-8667

BORDEAUX MODEL MANAGEMENT 616 N ROBERTSON BLVD LOS ANGELES CA 90069 (310) 289-2550

BORHMAN AGENCY 8489 W 3RD ST LOS ANGELES CA 90048 (213) 653-6701

BRAVERMAN GEKIS & BLOOM 6399 WILSHIRE BLVD LOS ANGELES CA 90048 (213) 782-4900

BUZZ HALLIDAY & ASSN 8899 BEVERLY BLVD LOS ANGELES CA 90048 (310) 275-6028

C'LA VIE MODEL & TALENT 7507 W SUNSET BLVD # 201 LOS ANGELES CA 90046 (213) 969-0541

CARLOS ALVARADO AGENCY 8455 BEVERLY BLVD LOS ANGELES CA 90048 (213) 655-7978

CARTER WRIGHT TALENT 6513 HOLLYWOOD BLVD # 210 LOS ANGELES CA 90028 (213) 469-0944

CASSELL LEVY INC 843 N SYCAMORE AVE LOS ANGELES CA 90038 (213) 461-3971

CAVALERI & ASSOC 849 S BROADWAY LOS ANGELES CA 90014 (213) 683-1354

CELEBRITY LOOK-ALIKES 7060 HOLLYWOOD BLVD # 1215 LOS ANGELES CA 90028 (213) 272-2006

CHARISMA MODEL MANAGEMENT 7060 HOLLYWOOD BLVD LOS ANGELES CA 90028 (213) 465-3960

CHARLES H STERN AGENCY INC 11766 WILSHIRE BLVD LOS ANGELES CA 90025 (310) 479-1788

CHARTER MANAGEMENT 1200 SANTEE ST LOS ANGELES CA 90015 (213) 745-3845

CHASIN AGENCY 8899 BEVERLY BLVD # 718 LOS ANGELES CA 90048 (310) 278-7505

CHATEAU BILLINGS 5657 WILSHIRE BLVD LOS ANGELES CA 90036 (213) 965-5432

CHL ARTISTS MANAGEMENT 1054 S ROBERTSON BLVD LOS ANGELES CA 90035 (310) 659-0800

CHN INTL AGENCY 7428 SANTA MONICA BLVD LOS ANGELES CA 90046 (213) 874-8252

CHRIS APODACA AGENCY 2049 E CENTURY PARK # 1200 LOS ANGELES CA 90067 (310) 284-3484

CITRUS GROUP 802 N CITRUS AVE LOS ANGELES CA 90038 (213) 466-8186

CLARK BRANSON 600 MOULTON AVE LOS ANGELES CA 90031 (213) 221-5894

*CLICK MODELS OF LOS ANGELES 9057 NEMO ST LOS ANGELES CA 90069 (310) 246-0800

CNA & ASSOC 1925 E CENTURY PARK # 750 LOS ANGELES CA 90067 (310) 556-4343

COLOURS INTERNATIONAL MODEL 8344 W 3RD ST # A LOS ANGELES CA 90048 (213) 658-7072

COLUMBUS & CO MANAGEMENT 10850 WILSHIRE BLVD LOS ANGELES CA 90024 (310) 441-2467

COSDEN AGENCY 3518 CAHUENGA BLVD W LOS ANGELES CA 90068 (213) 874-7200

CRAIG AGENCY 8485 MELROSE PL LOS ANGELES CA 90069 (213) 655-0236

CREATIVE PARTNERS 5750 WILSHIRE BLVD LOS ANGELES CA 90036 (213) 965-2581

CREW MEN AGENCY 8344 W 3RD ST # A LOS ANGELES CA 90048 (213) 658-7280

*CUNNINGHAM ESCOTT DIPENE 10635 SANTA MONICA BLVD LOS ANGELES CA 90025 (310) 475-3336

D H TALENT 1800 N HIGHLAND AVE LOS ANGELES CA 90028 (213) 962-6643

DAIMLER ARTIST AGENCY 2007 WILSHIRE BLVD LOS ANGELES CA 90057 (213) 483-9783

DALE GARRICK INTL AGENTS 8831 W SUNSET BLVD LOS ANGELES CA 90069 (310) 657-2661

DANA SNYDER TALENT 10641 LA GRANGE AVE LOS ANGELES CA 90025 (310) 441-0636

DANIEL BEN-AV PRODUCTIONS 9200 W SUNSET BLVD # 1220 LOS ANGELES CA 90069 (310) 271-5171

DEE'S KIDS & SENIOR CITIZEN 303 S CRESCENT HEIGHTS BLVD LOS ANGELES CA 90048 (213) 651-1066

DZA TALENT 8981 W SUNSET BLVD LOS ANGELES CA 90069 (310) 274-8025

EDGE MANAGEMENT 454 S ROBERTSON BLVD LOS ANGELES CA 90048 (310) 276-4049

EFENDI 1923 WESTWOOD BLVD # A LOS ANGELES CA 90025 (310) 441-2822

EFENDI AGENCY 6525 W SUNSET BLVD LOS ANGELES CA 90028 (213) 957-0006

ELAINE CRAIG CASTING 6565 W SUNSET BLVD LOS ANGELES CA 90028 (213) 469-8773

ERIK-MAGRATH CO 8833 W SUNSET BLVD LOS ANGELES CA 90069 (310) 854-6422

FARJA PRODUCTIONS 8929 S SEPULVEDA BLVD LOS ANGELES CA 90045 (310) 216-7769

FIERRO 803 N MANSFIELD AVE LOS ANGELES CA 90038 (213) 464-3148

FILM ARTISTS ASSOC 7080 HOLLYWOOD BLVD # 1118 LOS ANGELES CA 90028 (213) 463-1010

FINESSE MODEL MANAGEMENT 8250 W 3RD ST # 205 LOS ANGELES CA 90048 (213) 658-8269

FLASHCAST 3575 W CAHUENGA BLVD # 120 LOS ANGELES CA 90068 (818) 760-7986

FREELANCE MODELS 3575 CAHUENGA BLVD W LOS ANGELES CA 90068 (213) 850-3384

GAGE GROUP INC 9255 W SUNSET BLVD # 515 LOS ANGELES CA 90069 (310) 859-8777

GEDDES AGENCY 1203 GREENACRE AVE LOS ANGELES CA 90046 (213) 878-1155

GEORGE JAY TALENT AGENCY 6269 SELMA AVE # 15 LOS ANGELES CA 90028 (213) 466-6665

GERLER AGENCY 3349 W CAHUENGA BLVD # 1 LOS ANGELES CA 90068 (213) 850-7386

HALMARTER ENTERPRISES INC 3870 CRENSHAW BLVD LOS ANGELES CA 90008 (213) 298-1013

HALPERN & ASSOC 12304 SANTA MONICA BLVD LOS ANGELES CA 90025 (310) 571-4488

HANDS ON MANAGEMENT 8117 W SUNSET BLVD LOS ANGELES CA 90046 (213) 654-0943

HELEN GARRETT TALENT AGENCY 6525 W SUNSET BLVD LOS ANGELES CA 90028 (213) 871-8707

HENRY ONG MANAGEMENT 6362 HOLLYWOOD BLVD LOS ANGELES CA 90028 (213) 461-5699

HERB TANNEN & ASSOC 1800 VINE ST LOS ANGELES CA 90028 (213) 466-6191

HIGH PROFILE MANAGEMENT 7060 HOLLYWOOD BLVD LOS ANGELES CA 90028 (213) 462-1653

HWA TALENT REPRESENTATIVES 1964 WESTWOOD BLVD # 400 LOS ANGELES CA 90025 (310) 446-1313

INGENUE MODELS 3575 CAHUENGA BLVD W LOS ANGELES CA 90068 (213) 850-3322

INNOVATIVE ARTISTS TALENT 1999 AVENUE THE STARS LOS ANGELES CA 90067 (310) 553-5200

INNOVATIVE TALENT INC 8380 MELROSE AVE LOS ANGELES CA 90069 (213) 653-1363

INTERNATIONAL ARTS ENTR 10390 SANTA MONICA BLVD # 220 LOS ANGELES CA 90025 (310) 551-0014

INTERNATIONAL CASTING STUDIO 7060 HOLLYWOOD BLVD LOS ANGELES CA 90028 (213) 462-1656

*IT KIDS 526 N LARCHMONT BLVD LOS ANGELES CA 90004 (213) 962-5423

*IT MODEL MANAGEMENT 526 N LARCHMONT BLVD LOS ANGELES CA 90004 (213) 962-9564

*IT TALENT 526 N LARCHMONT BLVD LOS ANGELES CA 90004 (213) 962-5880

*J MICHAEL BLOOM & ASSOC LTD 957 COLE AVE LOS ANGELES CA 90038 (213) 465-9800

JEROME SIEGEL ASSOC 7551 W SUNSET BLVD # 203 LOS ANGELES CA 90046 (213) 850-1275

JOAN GREEN MANAGEMENT 8033 W SUNSET BLVD # 4048 LOS ANGELES CA 90046 (213) 878-0484

JOSEPH HELDFOND & RIX 1717 N HIGHLAND AVE LOS ANGELES CA 90028 (213) 466-9111

KELLEY KALLS 1800 N HIGHLAND AVE LOS ANGELES CA 90028 (213) 871-0098

KELMAN-ARLETTA 7813 W SUNSET BLVD LOS ANGELES CA 90046 (213) 851-8822

KEN LINDNER & ASSOC 2049 E CENTURY PARK # 2750 LOS ANGELES CA 90067 (310) 277-9223

KOMMY CORP OF AMERICA INC 630 N DOHENY DR LOS ANGELES CA 90069 (310) 278-9207

KRAGEN & CO 1112 N SHERBOURNE DR LOS ANGELES CA 90069 (310) 854-4400

*L A MODELS 8335 W SUNSET BLVD LOS ANGELES CA 90069 (213) 656-9572

*L A TALENT 8335 W SUNSET BLVD LOS ANGELES CA 90069 (213) 656-3722

LAWRENCE AGENCY 3575 W CAHUENGA BLVD # 125 LOS ANGELES CA 90068 (213) 851-7711

LEAVE HOME BOOKING 569 N ROSSMORE AVE LOS ANGELES CA 90004 (213) 856-9082

LESLIE ALLAN-RICE MANAGEMENT 7924 HILLSIDE AVE LOS ANGELES CA 90046 (213) 851-3364

LYONS & SHELDON AGENCY 8344 MELROSE AVE LOS ANGELES CA 90069 (213) 655-5100

MARION ROSENBERG OFC 8428 MELROSE PL LOS ANGELES CA 90069 (213) 653-7383

MARK JONES GROUP 1680 VINE ST # 802 LOS ANGELES CA 90028 (213) 462-4994

MARTEL AGENCY 1680 VINE ST LOS ANGELES CA 90028 (213) 461-5943

MC CONKEY ARTISTS AGENCY 1822 WILCOX AVE LOS ANGELES CA 90028 (213) 463-7141

METROPOLITAN TALENT AGENCY 4526 WILSHIRE BLVD LOS ANGELES CA 90010 (213) 857-4500

MICHAEL LIEN CASTING 7461 BEVERLY BLVD LOS ANGELES CA 90036 (213) 937-0411

MICHAEL SLESSENGER & ASSOC 8730 W SUNSET BLVD # 270 LOS ANGELES CA 90069 (310) 657-7113

MIRAMAR TALENT 7400 BEVERLY BLVD # 220 LOS ANGELES CA 90036 (310) 858-1900

MODEL CALL MAGAZINE 3575 CAHUENGA BLVD W LOS ANGELES CA 90068 (213) 850-3388

MODEL'S NETWORK 860 VINE ST LOS ANGELES CA 90038 (213) 463-3712

MODELS GUILD OF CALIFORNIA 7033 W SUNSET BLVD LOS ANGELES CA 90028 (213) 462-6861

MODELS' SUPPLIES & SVC BTQ 3575 CAHUENGA BLVD W LOS ANGELES CA 90068 (213) 851-3383

MOORE ARTIST TALENT AGENCY 1551 S ROBERTSON BLVD LOS ANGELES CA 90035 (310) 286-3150

MORE MEDAVOY MANAGEMENT 7920 W SUNSET BLVD LOS ANGELES CA 90046 (213) 969-0700

MUSE AGENCY 6100 WILSHIRE BLVD LOS ANGELES CA 90048 (213) 954-8968

NEW TALENT ENTERPRISES 2138 N CAHUENGA BLVD LOS ANGELES CA 90068 (213) 465-3365

NOBLE GROUP 3941 CUMBERLAND AVE LOS ANGELES CA 90027 (213) 665-9316

OTTO MODEL MANAGEMENT 1460 N. SWEETZER LOS ANGELES CA 90069 (213) 650-2200

P FAGEN PRODUCTIONS 1680 VINE ST LOS ANGELES CA 90028 (213) 465-6029

PACIFIC MANAGEMENT SVC 2774 LA CASTANA DR LOS ANGELES CA 90046 (213) 874-9559

PARADIGM 10100 SANTA MONICA BLVD # 25 LOS ANGELES CA 90067 (310) 277-4400

PETER STRAIN & ASSOC 8428 MELROSE PL LOS ANGELES CA 90069 (213) 782-8910

PETITE MODEL & TALENT MGMT 8360 MELROSE AVE LOS ANGELES CA 90069 (213) 782-9582

PLATINUM GROUP 10100 SANTA MONICA BLVD # 600 LOS ANGELES CA 90067 (310) 278-1535

PRIMA MANAGEMENT INC 933 N LA BREA AVE # 200 LOS ANGELES CA 90038 (213) 882-6900

PRIVILEGE TALENT 8170 BEVERLY BLVD LOS ANGELES CA 90048 (213) 658-8781

RICHARD POIRIER MODELS 3575 CAHUENGA BLVD W LOS ANGELES CA 90068 (213) 850-3380

ROBERT COSDEN ENTERPRISES 3518 W CAHUENGA BLVD # 216 LOS ANGELES CA 90068 (818) 752-4000

ROBERTS CO 10345 W OLYMPIC BLVD LOS ANGELES CA 90064 (310) 552-7800

SANDERS AGENCY LTD 8831 W SUNSET BLVD LOS ANGELES CA 90069 (310) 652-1119

SANDERS-KING MANAGEMENT 2211 CORINTH AVE LOS ANGELES CA 90064 (310) 312-5522

SANDIE SCHNARR TALENT 8281 MELROSE AVE # 200 LOS ANGELES CA 90046 (213) 653-9479

SARA BENNETT AGENCY 6404 HOLLYWOOD BLVD # 316 LOS ANGELES CA 90028 (213) 965-9666

SAVAGE AGENCY 6212 BANNER AVE LOS ANGELES CA 90038 (213) 461-8316

SCHIOWITZ CLAY ROSE INC 1680 VINE ST LOS ANGELES CA 90028 (213) 463-7300

SCOTT MANAGEMENT 8033 W SUNSET BLVD # 1200 LOS ANGELES CA 90046 (213) 856-4826

SDB PARTNERS INC 1801 AVENUE THE STARS LOS ANGELES CA 90067 (310) 785-0060

SHAPIRO-LICHTMAN INC 8827 BEVERLY BLVD LOS ANGELES CA 90048 (310) 859-8877

SHIRLEY WILSON & ASSOC 5410 WILSHIRE BLVD LOS ANGELES CA 90036 (213) 857-6977

SILVER MASSETTI & ASSOC 8730 W SUNSET BLVD # 480 LOS ANGELES CA 90069 (310) 289-0909

SMLA 8060 MELROSE AVE LOS ANGELES CA 90046 (213) 782-8999

SONNY MILLER AGENCY 6223 SELMA AVE # 101 LOS ANGELES CA 90028 (818) 845-6651

STUDIO ONE INTL 6565 W SUNSET BLVD LOS ANGELES CA 90028 (213) 957-1999

SUN AGENCY 8961 W SUNSET BLVD LOS ANGELES CA 90069 (310) 888-8737

SUNSET WEST TALENT AGENCY 8490 W SUNSET BLVD LOS ANGELES CA 90069 (310) 659-5340

SUSAN NATHE & ASSOC 8281 MELROSE AVE LOS ANGELES CA 90046 (213) 653-7573

SUTTON BARTH & VENNARI INC 145 S FAIRFAX AVE # 310 LOS ANGELES CA 90036 (213) 938-6000

TALENT HOUSE 7211 SANTA MONICA BLVD LOS ANGELES CA 90046 (213) 883-0360

TALENT MANAGEMENT ASSOC 326 N ORANGE DR LOS ANGELES CA 90036 (213) 937-3891

TEPPER-GALLEGOS CASTING 611 N LARCHMONT BLVD LOS ANGELES CA 90004 (213) 469-3577

TERRY BERLAND CASTING 12166 W OLYMPIC BLVD LOS ANGELES CA 90064 (310) 571-4141

TISHERMAN AGENCY INC 6767 FOREST LAWN DR LOS ANGELES CA 90068 (213) 850-6767

TLC BOOTH INC 6521 HOMEWOOD AVE LOS ANGELES CA 90028 (213) 464-2788

UMOJA TALENT AGENCY 2069 W SLAUSON AVE LOS ANGELES CA 90047 (213) 290-6612

VICTOR KRUGLOV & ASSOC 7060 HOLLYWOOD BLVD # 1220 LOS ANGELES CA 90028 (213) 957-9000

W RANDOLPH CLARK CO 2431 HYPERION AVE LOS ANGELES CA 90027 (213) 953-4960

WESTSIDE CASTING 12166 W OLYMPIC BLVD LOS ANGELES CA 90064 (310) 820-9200

WILD BRIAR TALENT 1608 N CAHUENGA BLVD LOS ANGELES CA 90028 (213) 850-8136

WILLIAM FELBER AGENCY 2126 N CAHUENGA BLVD LOS ANGELES CA 90068 (213) 466-7626

WILLIAM KERWIN AGENCY 1605 N CAHUENGA BLVD # 202 LOS ANGELES CA 90028 (213) 469-5155

WORLD MANAGEMENT 2040 AVENUE THE STARS LOS ANGELES CA 90067 (310) 277-0100

ABRA EDELMAN CASTING 16170 KENNEDY RD LOS GATOS CA 95032 (408) 356-2804

PATRICIA LITTLE & CO 127 GALLEON ST MARINA DEL REY CA 90292 (310) 305-1820

SUPER TALENT AGENCY RESOURCES 655 REDWOOD HWY MILL VALLEY CA 94941 (415) 479-7827

RENDE MODELS 726 14TH ST MODESTO CA 95354 (209) 526-6881

ARTIST MANAGEMENT AGENCY 4340 CAMPUS DR # 210 NEWPORT BEACH CA 92660 (714) 261-7557

FLORENCE SMALES MODEL AGENCY 2110 VISTA LAREDO NEWPORT BEACH CA 92660 (714) 759-3143

JUDY VENN & ASSOC 1500 QUAIL ST # 260 NEWPORT BEACH CA 92660 (714) 975-1664

KIDS HOLLYWOOD CONNECTION 1151 DOVE ST # 225 NEWPORT BEACH CA 92660 (714) 851-0920

TALENT SHOP 1539 MONROVIA AVE NEWPORT BEACH CA 92663 (714) 722-9720

ANN WAUGH TALENT 4741 LAUREL CANYON BLVD NORTH HOLLYWOOD CA 91607 (818) 980-0141

BIGLEY TALENT 6442 COLDWATER CYN AVE # 211 NORTH HOLLYWOOD CA 91606 (818) 761-9978

CINDY OSBRINK PRINT KIDS 4605 LANKERSHIM BLVD NORTH HOLLYWOOD CA 91602 (818) 760-2803

CINDY OSBRINK TALENT 4605 LANKERSHIM BLVD # 401 NORTH HOLLYWOOD CA 91602 (818) 760-2488

COAST TO COAST TALENT GROUP 4942 VINELAND AVE NORTH HOLLYWOOD CA 91601 (818) 762-6278

CORALIE JR THEATRICAL AGENCY 4789 VINELAND AVE NORTH HOLLYWOOD CA 91602 (818) 766-9501

GORES-FIELDS AGENCY 10443 KLING ST NORTH HOLLYWOOD CA 91602 (818) 508-8945

JACK SCAGNETTI TALENT AGENCY 5118 VINELAND AVE NORTH HOLLYWOOD CA 91601 (818) 761-0580

KATIE'S KIDS 4605 LANKERSHIM BLVD NORTH HOLLYWOOD CA 91602 (818) 761-0611

LUND AGENCY INDUSTRY ARTIST 10000 RIVERSIDE DR NORTH HOLLYWOOD CA 91602 (818) 508-1688

MARY GRADY AGENCY 4444 LANKERSHIM BLVD # 207 NORTH HOLLYWOOD CA 91602 (818) 766-4414

MODEL TEAM 12435 OXNARD ST NORTH HOLLYWOOD CA 91606 (818) 755-0026

MODELS NETWORK 4741 LAUREL CANYON BLVD NORTH HOLLYWOOD CA 91607 (818) 769-0920

MULTI TALENT INC 6156 SIMPSON AVE NORTH HOLLYWOOD CA 91606 (818) 766-5192

PATTY MITCHELL AGENC 4605 LANKERSHIM BLVD # 201 NORTH HOLLYWOOD CA 91602 (818) 508-6181

SCREEN ARTIST AGENCY 12435 OXNARD ST NORTH HOLLYWOOD CA 91606 (818) 755-0026

TYLER KJAR AGENCY 10643 RIVERSIDE DR NORTH HOLLYWOOD CA 91602 (818) 760-0321

WHITAKER AGENCY 4924 VINELAND AVE NORTH HOLLYWOOD CA 91601 (818) 766-4441

YOUNG ARTISTS MANAGEMNT 4739 LANKERSHIM BLVD NORTH HOLLYWOOD CA 91602 (818) 985-6834

CREATIVE ARTIST MANAGEMENT 436 14TH ST OAKLAND CA 94612 (510) 451-5351

PETERSON & ASSOC 1404 FRANKLIN ST OAKLAND CA 94612 (510) 444-3424

LIANA FIELDS TALENT AGENCY 2181 S EL CAMINO REAL OCEANSIDE CA 92054 (619) 433-6429

PARADISE ARTISTS 108 E MATILIJA ST OJAI CA 93023 (805) 646-8433

LACEY & ASSOC 1550 N CASE ST ORANGE CA 92867 (714) 660-1001

SAXON MODEL & TALENT 777 S MAIN ST ORANGE CA 92868 (714) 836-1694

BURSTEIN CO 520 SALERNO DR PACIFIC PLSDS CA 90272 (310) 454-9462

CINDY ROMANO MODELING 414 VILLAGE SQ W PALM SPRINGS CA 92262 (619) 346-1694

CINDY ROMANO MODELING 266 S PALM CANYON DR PALM SPRINGS CA 92262 (619) 323-3333

DOROTHY SHREVE SCHOOL 2665 N PALM CANYON DR PALM SPRINGS CA 92262 (619) 327-5855

MADLIN'S MODELING AGENCY 2688 E JULIAN RD PALM SPRINGS CA 92262 (619) 327-3060

PALM SPRINGS EXTRA 227 RAINCLOUD ST PALM SPRINGS CA 92264 (619) 325-8888

SEBSTIAN GIBSON AGENCY 125 E TAHQUITZ CANYON WAY PALM SPRINGS CA 92262 (619) 322-2200

KISER MODELS 37348 LARAMIE ST PALMDALE CA 93552 (805) 285-2535

AGENCY FOR TALENT 750 E GREEN ST PASADENA CA 91101 (818) 795-7651

INTERNATIONAL MODEL MNGMNT 235 E COLORADO BLVD, #244 PASADENA CA 91101 (818) 796-4525

WALTER TRASK THEATRICAL AGENCY 750 E GREEN ST PASADENA CA 91101 (213) 681-3766

WEST COAST MODELS 1610 OAK PARK BLVD PLEASANT HILL CA 94523 (510) 932-6774

MONTGOMERY MANAGEMENT TALENT 981 HOPKINS WAY PLEASANTON CA 94566 (510) 417-7480

A CLASS ACT MODELING 2950 BECHELLI LN REDDING CA 96002 (916) 222-3111

MITCHELL MODELS INTL 225 AVENUE I # 204 REDONDO BEACH CA 90277 (310) 792-9040

PACIFIC TALENT & MODELS 1914 S PACIFIC COAST HWY REDONDO BEACH CA 90277 (310) 543-1018

ALPHA TALENT 2395 EL CAMINO AVE SACRAMENTO CA 95821 (916) 972-9991

CARUSO & CO 1610 ARDEN WAY SACRAMENTO CA 95815 (916) 921-1564

CAST IMAGES 1125 FIREHOUSE ALY SACRAMENTO CA 95814 (916) 444-9720

NORTHERN CALIFORNIA CASTING 3411 ARDEN WAY SACRAMENTO CA 95825 (916) 488-4517

TALENT MARKETING 77 CADILLAC DR # 188 SACRAMENTO CA 95825 (916) 565-4700

J P CLYMER'S MODELING & TALENT 649 SAN ANSELMO AVE SAN ANSELMO CA 94960 (415) 457-5845

PENNY CLYMER & CO 649 SAN ANSELMO AVE SAN ANSELMO CA 94960 (415) 457-7726

BARBIZON SCHOOL OF MODELING 636 E BRIER DR # 150 SAN BERNARDINO CA 92408 (909) 884-6266

AGENCY 2 MODEL & TALENT AGENCY 2425 SAN DIEGO AVE # 211 SAN DIEGO CA 92110 (619) 291-9556

ANDY ANDERSON TALENT AGENCY 7801 MISSION CTR SAN DIEGO CA 92108 (619) 294-4629

ARTIST MANAGEMENT AGENCY 835 5TH AVE # 411 SAN DIEGO CA 92101 (619) 233-6655

AVANTI TALENT & PRODUCTION SVC 2870 5TH AVE # 3 SAN DIEGO CA 92103 (619) 295-4900

JANICE PATTERSON AGENCY 2254 MOORE ST # 104 SAN DIEGO CA 92110 (619) 295-9477

NOUVEAU MODEL TALENT MGMT 2801 CAMINO DEL RIO S SAN DIEGO CA 92108 (619) 295-4500

NOUVEAU NEW FACES DEV CTR 2801 S CAMINO DEL RIO # 300 SAN DIEGO CA 92108 (619) 453-2727

PRECISE TALENT AGENCY 4640 JEWELL ST # 230W SAN DIEGO CA 92109 (619) 270-9200

REGISTRY OF TALENT 5060 SHOREHAM PL SAN DIEGO CA 92122 (619) 622-8913

RKP MANAGEMENT GROUP PO BOX 710972 SAN DIEGO CA 92171 (619) 299-7464

SAN DIEGO MODEL MANAGEMENT 824 N CAMINO DEL RIO # 552 SAN DIEGO CA 92108 (619) 296-1018

SHAMON FREITAS MODEL & TAL 9606 TIERRA GRANDE STE 204 SAN DIEGO CA 92126 (619) 549-3955

TINA REAL CASTING 3108 5TH AVE SAN DIEGO CA 92103 (619) 298-0544

WATKINS TALENT MANAGEMENT 5440 MOREHOUSE DR SAN DIEGO CA 92121 (619) 622-6262

ADKISON MODEL MANAGEMENT 699 8TH ST # 3106 SAN FRANCISCO CA 94103 (415) 626-1183

ALANDREAS FASHION-MODELS PO BOX 590172 SAN FRANCISCO CA 94159 (415) 754-1531

ANIMATION TALENT AGENCY 1282 SACRAMENTO ST SAN FRANCISCO CA 94108 (415) 776-7983

AVALON MODELS 166 GEARY ST # 1300 SAN FRANCISCO CA 94108 (415) 421-8211

BARBARA DAVIS MODELING SCHOOL 647 BRAZIL AVE SAN FRANCISCO CA 94112 (415) 239-1906

BARBIZON SCHOOL OF MODELING 447 SUTTER ST SAN FRANCISCO CA 94108 (415) 391-4254

BOOKINGS MODELS MANAGEMENT CO 870 MARKET ST SAN FRANCISCO CA 94102 (415) 296-9647

*BOOM MODELS & TALENT 2325 3RD ST, #223 SAN FRANCISCO CA 94107 (415) 626-6591

CHARLES WEITZER & ASSOC 166 GEARY ST SAN FRANCISCO CA 94108 (415) 391-4041

CITY MODEL & TALENT MNGMNT 123 TOWNSEND ST # 510 SAN FRANCISCO CA 94107 (415) 546-3160

EIKO'S AGENCY 150 POWELL ST SAN FRANCISCO CA 94102 (415) 398-8830

FILM-THEATRE-ACTORS EXCHANGE 582 MARKET ST SAN FRANCISCO CA 94104 (415) 433-3920

GENERATIONS MODEL & TALENT 350 TOWNSEND ST SAN FRANCISCO CA 94107 (415) 777-9099

JENNIFER SPALDING & ASSOC 1728 UNION ST SAN FRANCISCO CA 94123 (415) 346-6177

KIDS ON CAMERA TV ACTING SCHL 84 1ST ST SAN FRANCISCO CA 94105 (415) 882-9878

LOOK MODEL AGENCY 166 GEARY ST # 1400 SAN FRANCISCO CA 94108 (415) 781-2822

LOOK MODEL-CHILDREN & INFO 166 GEARY ST SAN FRANCISCO CA 94108 (415) 781-5665

*MARLA DELL TALENT 2124 UNION ST SAN FRANCISCO CA 94123 (415) 563-9213

MITCHELL TALENT MANAGEMENT 323 GEARY ST # 302 SAN FRANCISCO CA 94102 (415) 395-9291

PALMER'S MODEL & TALENT AGENCY 699 8TH ST # 3260A SAN FRANCISCO CA 94103 (415) 553-4100

PRESTIGE MODEL & TALENT MGMT 330 TOWNSEND ST SAN FRANCISCO CA 94107 (415) 543-2980

QUEUE AGENCY 66 MINT ST SAN FRANCISCO CA 94103 (415) 896-6962

QUINN-TONRY INC 601 BRANNAN ST SAN FRANCISCO CA 94107 (415) 543-3797

RAVE BOOKING AGENCY 3470 19TH ST SAN FRANCISCO CA 94110 (415) 865-2170

REVE AGENCY 699 8TH AVE SAN FRANCISCO CA 94118 (415) 621-6419

SUZANNE CLARK MODELING CONSLNT 25 VAN NESS AVE SAN FRANCISCO CA 94102 (415) 776-4900

TOP MODELS AND TALENT 870 MARKET ST # 1076 SAN FRANCISCO CA 94102 (415) 391-1800

FRAZER AGENCY 4300 STEVENS CREEK BLVD # 126 SAN JOSE CA 95129 (408) 554-1055

HALVORSON-FUNG MODEL MGMT 2858 STEVENS CREEK BLVD SAN JOSE CA 95128 (408) 983-1038

LOS LATINOS TALENT AGENCY 2801 MOORPARK AVE # 11 SAN JOSE CA 95128 (408) 296-2213

ON STAGE PRODUCTION TALENT 330 S BASCOM AVE SAN JOSE CA 95128 (408) 292-3684

T-BEST TALENT AGENCY 2001 WAYNE AVE SAN LEANDRO CA 94577 (510) 357-6865

SUSAN LANE MODEL & TALENT AGCY 14071 WINDSOR PL SANTA ANA CA 92705 (714) 731-7827

AGENTIA 1815 STATE ST SANTA BARBARA CA 93101 (805) 569-9588

CLASS ACT 1727 STATE ST SANTA BARBARA CA 93101 (805) 882-9289

INTEGRITY CASTING 1825 PRUNERIDGE AVE SANTA CLARA CA 95050 (408) 243-9466

THIERMANN DAVID S 1725 SEABRIGHT AVE SANTA CRUZ CA 95062 (408) 427-2677

CLOUTIER TALENT AGENCY 1026 MONTANA AVE SANTA MONICA CA 90403 (213) 931-1323

IMT 225 SANTA MONICA BLVD # 1005 SANTA MONICA CA 90401 (310) 260-0168

SCRIPT WORKS 2425 COLORADO AVE SANTA MONICA CA 90404 (310) 264-8255

STUDIO TALENT GROUP 1328 12TH ST SANTA MONICA CA 90401 (310) 393-8004

BELISSIMA MODELS 2142 VINTAGE CIR SANTA ROSA CA 95404 (707) 523-0819

COVERS MODEL & TALENT AGENCY 4716 FOULGER DR SANTA ROSA CA 95405 (707) 539-9252

PANDA TALENT AGENCY 3721 HOEN AVE SANTA ROSA CA 95405 (707) 576-0711

PARAGON ACADEMY 509 4TH ST SANTA ROSA CA 95401 (707) 579-8779

MODELING CONNECTION 12340 SARATOGA SUNNYVALE RD SARATOGA CA 95070 (408) 996-2001

A M ARTISTS MANAGEMENT 28306 EVERGREEN LN SAUGUS CA 91350 (805) 297-6111

MAIN STREET THEATRE 104 N MAIN ST SEBASTOPOL CA 95472 (707) 823-0177

APODACA & MUNRO TALENT AGENCY 13801 VENTURA BLVD SHERMAN OAKS CA 91423 (818) 380-2700

BARUCK-CONSOLO MANAGEMENT 15003 GREENLEAF ST SHERMAN OAKS CA 91403 (818) 907-9072

BEST AGENCY INC 13437 VENTURA BLVD SHERMAN OAKS CA 91423 (818) 783-9537

BIZ FOR KIDS PO BOX 56204 SHERMAN OAKS CA 91413 (818) 9097015

DAVID SHAPIRA & ASSOC 15301 VENTURA BLVD SHERMAN OAKS CA 91403 (818) 906-0322

KEN B JOHNSTON & ASSOC 15043 VALLEYHEART DR SHERMAN OAKS CA 91403 (213) 461-8257

LEVINE EVELYN 15233 VENTURA BLVD SHERMAN OAKS CA 91403 (213) 655-8968

NUSBAUM TALENT MANAGEMENT 13557 VENTURA BLVD # A SHERMAN OAKS CA 91423 (818) 784-6570

WORLD MODELING AGENCY 4523 VAN NUYS BLVD SHERMAN OAKS CA 91403 (818) 986-4316

ALLIED BOOKING CO-TALENT 2733 VIA ORANGE WAY # 104 SPRING VALLEY CA 91978 (619) 660-9111

ALPERN GROUP 4400 COLDWATER CANYON AVE STUDIO CITY CA 91604 (818) 752-1877

ARLENE THORNTON & ASSOC 12001 VENTURA PL STUDIO CITY CA 91604 (818) 760-6688

BEVERLY HECHT AGENCY 12001 VENTURA PL # 320 STUDIO CITY CA 91604 (310) 278-3544

CAREER ARTISTS INTL AGENCY 11030 VENTURA BLVD STUDIO CITY CA 91604 (818) 980-1315

DADE-SCHULTZ ASSOC 11846 VENTURA BLVD STUDIO CITY CA 91604 (818) 760-3100

DIANE DIMEO & ASSOC 12754 SARAH ST STUDIO CITY CA 91604 (818) 505-0945

FEATURE PLAYERS AGENCY 4051 RADFORD AVE STUDIO CITY CA 91604 (818) 508-6691

HERVEY GRIMES TALENT AGENCY 4518 MORSE AVE STUDIO CITY CA 91604 (818) 981-0891

HERVEY GRIMES TALENT AGENCY 12444 VENTURA BLVD STUDIO CITY CA 91604 (818) 980-3181

HOWARD TALENT WEST 12229 VENTURA BLVD STUDIO CITY CA 91604 (818) 766-5300

KAZARIAN SPENCER & ASSOC INC 11365 VENTURA BLVD STUDIO CITY CA 91604 (818) 769-9111

LAWRENCE RAY LTD PO BOX 1987 STUDIO CITY CA 91614 (818) 508-9022

MERIDIAN TALENT AGENCY 13223 VENTURA BLVD STUDIO CITY CA 91604 (818) 905-1516

NEWMAN-THOMAS MANAGEMENT 12403 VENTURA CT STUDIO CITY CA 91604 (818) 763-0567

OMNIPOP INC 10700 VENTURA BLVD STUDIO CITY CA 91604 (818) 980-9267

TERRY LICHTMAN CO 4439 WORTSER AVE STUDIO CITY CA 91604 (818) 783-3003

TURTLE AGENCY 12456 VENTURA BLVD # 1 STUDIO CITY CA 91604 (818) 506-6898

PEOPLE FINDERS 962 WESTCREEK LN # 232 THOUSAND OAKS CA 91362 (818) 706-7322

STAR TALENT 4555 MARIOTA AVE TOLUCA LAKE CA 91602 (818) 509-1931

ALESE MARSHALL MODEL 23900 HAWTHORNE BLVD TORRANCE CA 90505 (310) 378-1223

LITTLE MISS HAWAIIAN TROPIC 351 N WALNUT RD TURLOCK CA 95380 (209) 668-7969

*BOBBY BALL TALENT AGENCY 4342 LANKERSHIM BLVD UNIVERSAL CITY CA 91602 (818) 506-8188

WILMAR TALENT AGENCY 14329 VICTORY BLVD VAN NUYS CA 91401 (818) 781-8539

MARTA MICHAUD MANAGEMENT 28 S VENICE BLVD VENICE CA 90291 (310) 577-5878

ABRAMS ARTISTS & ASSOC 9200 W SUNSET BLVD WEST HOLLYWOOD CA 90069 (310) 859-0625

ADWATER & STIR INC 9000 W SUNSET BLVD WEST HOLLYWOOD CA 90069 (310) 970-1900

ANITA HAEGGSTROM AGENCY 8721 W SUNSET BLVD WEST HOLLYWOOD CA 90069 (310) 289-1071

BERNARD FELDMAN MANAGEMENT 8764 HOLLOWAY DR WEST HOLLYWOOD CA 90069 (310) 652-8181

DON BUCHWALD & ASSOC 9229 W SUNSET BLVD WEST HOLLYWOOD CA 90069 (310) 278-3600

FERRAR MAZIROFF ASSOC 8430 SANTA MONICA BLVD WEST HOLLYWOOD CA 90069 (213) 654-2601

GORDON RAEL CO 9255 W SUNSET BLVD WEST HOLLYWOOD CA 90069 (310) 285-9552

KRAFT AGENCY 1201 LARRABEE ST WEST HOLLYWOOD CA 90069 (310) 652-6065

KRAFT AGENCY INC 8491 W SUNSET BLVD # 492 WEST HOLLYWOOD CA 90069 (310) 652-6065

LOS ANGELES SPORTS 8439 W SUNSET BLVD WEST HOLLYWOOD CA 90069 (213) 654-4880

MARK SHIMMEL MANAGEMENT 8899 BEVERLY BLVD WEST HOLLYWOOD CA 90048 (818) 881-0090

MARY WEBB DAVIS AGENCY 515 N LA CIENEGA BLVD WEST HOLLYWOOD CA 90048 (213) 655-6747

MC GOWAN MANAGEMENT 8733 W SUNSET BLVD WEST HOLLYWOOD CA 90069 (310) 289-9157

MODEL'S EXCHANGE 8833 W SUNSET BLVD WEST HOLLYWOOD CA 90069 (310) 657-3203

*NEXT MANAGEMENT 662 N. ROBERTSON BLVD WEST HOLLYWOOD CA 90069 (310) 358-0100

NEXT MANAGEMENT CO 662 N ROBERTSON BLVD WEST HOLLYWOOD CA 90069 (310) 358-0100

PAKULA KING & ASSOC 9229 W SUNSET BLVD WEST HOLLYWOOD CA 90069 (310) 281-4868

PARAGON TALENT AGENCIES 8439 W SUNSET BLVD WEST HOLLYWOOD CA 90069 (213) 654-4245

PLAYERS TALENT AGENCY 8770 SHOREHAM DR WEST HOLLYWOOD CA 90069 (310) 289-8777

PTI TALENT MANAGEMENT 662 N ROBERTSON BLVD WEST HOLLYWOOD CA 90069 (310) 358-0100

TBS CASTING 8831 W SUNSET BLVD WEST HOLLYWOOD CA 90069 (310) 854-1955

VANGUARD TALENT MANAGEMENT 9200 W SUNSET BLVD WEST HOLLYWOOD CA 90069 (310) 777-0123

VICKI CLEMENCE MODELING CTR 14826 WHITTIER BLVD WHITTIER CA 90605 (310) 698-8861

A TOTAL ACTING EXPERIENCE 20501 VENTURA BLVD WOODLAND HILLS CA 91364 (818) 340-9249

COLORADO

TALENTIERING 6295 WADSWORTH BLVD ARVADA CO 80003 (303) 425-5641

CAST OF ASPEN 520 E COOPER ST ASPEN CO 81611 (970) 925-1357

JOHN ROBERT POWERS MODELING 14231 E 4TH AVE # 200 AURORA CO 80011 (303) 3402838

SILHOUETTES MODELING & ACTING 3980 BROADWAY ST BOULDER CO 80304 (303) 449-7765

JAC WINROTH ASSOC 10221 W 102ND AVE BROOMFIELD CO 80021 (303) 469-3313

ACTORS HAVEN 4827 BARNES RD COLORADO SPRINGS CO 80917 (719) 596-7471

ACTORS HAVEN 121 E PIKES PEAK AVE # 207 COLORADO SPRINGS CO 80903 (719) 471-4325

JEANINE'S MODELING & TALENT 1227 MOUNT VIEW LN COLORADO SPRINGS CO 80907 (719) 598-4507

MTA TALENT AGENCY 1026 W COLORADO AVE COLORADO SPRINGS CO 80904 (719) 577-4704

BARBIZON TALENT AGENCY 7535 E HAMPDEN AVE DENVER CO 80231 (303) 337-7954

BIG FISH TALENT REPRESENTATION 312 W 1ST AVE DENVER CO 80223 (303) 744-7170

DONNA BALDWIN TALENT INC 50 S STEELE ST # 260 DENVER CO 80209 (303) 320-0067

EDGE TALENT MANAGEMENT 1821 BLAKE ST DENVER CO 80202 (303) 685-4949

JOHN CASABLANCAS MODELING CTR 7600 E EASTMAN AVE DENVER CO 80231 (303) 337-5100

KIDSKITS INC 136 KALAMATH ST DENVER CO 80223 (303) 446-8200

MARBLES KIDS MANAGEMENT INC 240 JOSEPHINE ST # 205 DENVER CO 80206 (303) 322-5004

MAXIMUM TALENT INC 3900 E MEXICO AVE # 105 DENVER CO 80210 (303) 691-2344

MODEL & TALENT MANAGEMENT 7600 E EASTMAN AVE DENVER CO 80231 (303) 337-4541

SIEGEL REPRESENTS INC 1539 PLATTE ST # 205 DENVER CO 80202 (303) 722-3456

VOICE CHOICE 1805 S BELLAIRE ST DENVER CO 80222 (303) 756-9055

FIRST STAR 5650 GREENWOOD PLZ # 210 ENGLEWOOD CO 80111 (303) 694-3244

SILHOUETTES TALENT AGENCY 12892 W LOUISIANA AVE LAKEWOOD CO 80228 (303) 904-8485

ANDREE KIT TALENT INTL 3901 W 88TH AVE WESTMINSTER CO 80030 (303) 430-0060

LEITEN VIA-AGENCY 8704 YATES DR WESTMINSTER CO 80030 (303) 657-9105

VIA TALENT MARKETING 8704 YATES DR WESTMINSTER CO 80030 (303) 657-9105

CONNECTICUT

SCREEN TEST USA 700 W JOHNSON AVE CHESHIRE CT 06410 (203) 250-8268

GREENWICH MODEL GROUP 25 W ELM ST # 11 GREENWICH CT 06830 (203) 869-2772

JOHN CASABLANCAS MODELING CTR 461 FARMINGTON AVE HARTFORD CT 06105 (860) 232-4421

NEW ENGLAND'S CHILDREN MODELS 292 NEW BRITAIN RD KENSINGTON CT 06037 (860) 829-1365

CREATIVE TALENT LTD 66 LAUREL LN MARLBOROUGH CT 06447 (860) 295-1060

LELAS TALENT AGENCY 56 QUIRK RD MILFORD CT 06460 (203) 877-8355

JOHNSTON MODELING AGENCY 50 WASHINGTON ST NORWALK CT 06854 (203) 838-6188

BARBIZON SCHOOL OF MODELING 26 6TH ST # 301 STAMFORD CT 06905 (203) 359-0427

CURTAIN CALL 1349 NEWFIELD AVE STAMFORD CT 06905 (203) 329-8207

CHILDRENS PROFESSIONAL SCHOOL 5859 MAIN ST TRUMBULL CT 06611 (203) 268-9550

ALLISON DANIELS MODEL MGMT 1260 NEW BRITAIN AVE WEST HARTFORD CT 06110 (860) 561-4483

JOANNA LAWRENCE AGENCY 82 PARTRICK RD WESTPORT CT 06880 (203) 226-7239

NEWSTAR INC 55 GRISWOLD RD WETHERSFIELD CT 06109 (860) 529-7761

VISAGE MODELS INC 87 COLTON ST WINDSOR CT 06095 (860) 525-9800

WASHINGTON, D.C.

ANNE SCHWAB'S MODEL STORE 1529 WISCONSIN AVE NW WASHINGTON DC 20007 (202) 333-3560

ARTIST AGENCY 3070 M ST NW WASHINGTON DC 20007 (202) 342-0933

CAPITAL CASTING 1937 BILTMORE ST NW WASHINGTON DC 20009 (202) 797-8621

CENTRAL CASTING INC 623 PENNSYLVANIA AVE SE WASHINGTON DC 20003 (202) 547-6300

DORAN MODELS & TALENTS 1404 27TH ST NW WASHINGTON DC 20007 (202) 333-6367

SHAKESPEARE THEATRE 301 E CAPITOL ST SE WASHINGTON DC 20003 (202) 547-3230

STARS CASTING 1301 NW 20TH ST # 101 WASHINGTON DC 20036 (202) 429-9494

DELAWARE

BARBIZON SCHOOL OF MODELING 17 TROLLEY SQ WILMINGTON DE 19806 (302) 658-6666

CNH TALENT CTR 1719 DELAWARE AVE WILMINGTON DE 19806 (302) 425-5915

CREATIVE IMAGES MODELING SCHL 222 PHILADELPHIA PIKE WILMINGTON DE 19809 (302) 764-9514

FLORIDA

BROADWAY MODELING & TALENT 249 W STATE RD 436 ALTAMONTE SPGS FL 32714 (407) 869-1144

OMNI TALENT GROUP INC 101 S WYMORE RD # 405 ALTAMONTE SPGS FL 32714 (407) 774-6664

ELLE MODELS INC 1199 S FEDERAL HWY BOCA RATON FL 33432 (561) 361-9988

SCREEN TEST USA 5301 N FEDERAL HWY BOCA RATON FL 33487 (561) 998-3790

ELLEN MEADE STUDIOS 1323 63RD AVE E BRADENTON FL 34203 (941) 755-1757

A A ARTISTS INC 30 COTILLION CT CASSELBERRY FL 32707 (407) 339-3612

ALL STAR MODELS & TALENT 30 COTILLION CT CASSELBERRY FL 32707 (407) 339-3612

ARIZA TALENT & MODELING AGENCY 909 STATE RD 436 CASSELBERRY FL 32707 (407) 332-0011

ASHLEY CAMILLE SCHOOL OF IMAGE 909 SEMORAN BLVD CASSELBERRY FL 32707 (407) 332-0195

CREATIVE TALENT MANAGEMENT INC 2561 NURSERY RD CLEARWATER FL 34624 (813) 532-3992

HAMILTON-HALL TALENT INC 13700 58TH ST N CLEARWATER FL 34620 (813) 538-3838

JO'S INTERNATIONAL MODELS INC 4500 140TH AVE N CLEARWATER FL 34622 (813) 535-0520

ANNE O'BRIANT AGENCY INC 1260 FRAN MAR CT CLERMONT FL 34711 (352) 242-9983

ELVA'S TALENT AGENCY 717 PONCE DE LEON BLVD CORAL GABLES FL 33134 (305) 444-9071

JOBS & MODELS UNLIMITED 337 8TH ST DAYTONA BEACH FL 32117 (904) 253-6730

BOCA MODELS 829 SE 9TH ST DEERFIELD BEACH FL 33441 (954) 428-4677

A-1 PEG'S TALENT & MODELING 133 E LAUREN CT FERN PARK FL 32730 (407) 834-0406

AARON MODEL & TALENT 2803 E COMMERCIAL BLVD FORT LAUDERDALE FL 33308 (954) 772-8944

ANGEL INTERNATN'L MNGMT 2101 W COMMERCIAL BLVD FORT LAUDERDALE FL 33309 (954) 676-5555

AVENUE PRODUCTIONS 2810 E OAKLAND PARK BLVD # 308 FORT LAUDERDALE FL 33306 (954) 561-2187

JACQUES MODELS INC 2440 E COMMERCIAL BLVD # 4 FORT LAUDERDALE FL 33308 (954) 938-7226

JOHN CASABLANCAS 3343 W COMMERCIAL BLVD # 106 FORT LAUDERDALE FL 33309 (954) 731-6333

MARIAN POLAN TALENT AGENCY 10 NE 11TH AVE FORT LAUDERDALE FL 33301 (954) 525-8351

MODEL'S EXCHANGE 2425 E COMMERCIAL BLVD # 206 FORT LAUDERDALE FL 33308 (954) 491-4266

PATTI BOOKOUT & ASSOC 2767 E SUNRISE BLVD FORT LAUDERDALE FL 33304 (954) 561-2333

SCOTT HARVEY MODEL & 2734 E OAKLAND PARK BLVD FORT LAUDERDALE FL 33306 (954) 565-1211

SHOWMASTERS 3038 N FEDERAL HWY FORT LAUDERDALE FL 33306 (954) 563-8028

SMITH & BAKER PROMO AGCY 2455 E SUNRISE BLVD FORT LAUDERDALE FL 33304 (954) 568-5942

STAGE LEFT PRODUCTIONS 10062 NW 46TH ST FORT LAUDERDALE FL 33351 (954) 747-7474

FIRESTONE MODELING 31 BARKLEY CIR # 1 FORT MYERS FL 33907 (941) 939-3880

FIRESTONE SCHOOL OF MODELING 31 BARKLEY CIR FORT MYERS FL 33907 (941) 939-3918

LONGSHOT TALENT AGENCY 1483 SAUTERN DR FORT MYERS FL 33919 (941) 433-0248

TAKE ONE CASTING 8695 COLLEGE PKY FORT MYERS FL 33919 (941) 945-3033

MARY LOU'S MODEL MANGMNT 446 RACETRACK RD NW FORT WALTON BCH FL 32547 (904) 862-1004

*FLORIDA STARS MODEL & TALENT 225 W UNIVERSITY AVE GAINESVILLE FL 32601 (352) 338-1086

PIERRE BLANCHET & ASSOC 4445 SW 35TH TER # 110 GAINESVILLE FL 32608 (352) 377-0581

*MARY LOU'S MODELS 913 GULF BREEZE PKY # 15 GULF BREEZE FL 32561 (904) 939-3204

J B MONROE INC 2991 SW 32ND AVE HOLLYWOOD FL 33023 (954) 986-9433

*DENISE CAROL MODELS & TALENT 3236 BEACH BLVD JACKSONVILLE FL 32207 (904) 399-0824

JOHN CASABLANCAS STUDIOS 8380 BAYMEADOWS RD # 14 JACKSONVILLE FL 32256 (904) 739-1118

MISS PONTE VEDRA BEACH INC 8833 COVENTRY CT JACKSONVILLE FL 32257 (904) 448-6927

MODEL & TALENT MANAGEMENT 8380 BAYMEADOWS RD # 14 JACKSONVILLE FL 32256 (904) 739-0619

PERSONAL PROFILE MODELING AGCY 7530 103RD ST JACKSONVILLE FL 32210 (904) 573-7980

SELECT MODELS & TALENT 5991 CHESTER AVE JACKSONVILLE FL 32217 (904) 730-2046

*SESSIONS MODELING STUDIO 8258 ARLINGTON EXPY JACKSONVILLE FL 32211 (904) 724-3101

*IRENE MARIE INC 728 OCEAN DR KEY BISCAYNE FL 33149 (305) 672-2929

*CHRISTENSEN TALENT GROUP 120 INTERNATIONAL PKY # 262 LAKE MARY FL 32746 (407) 628-8803

STELLA JAY BROWN MODELING INC 605 YORKTOWN DR LEESBURG FL 34748 (352) 787-7004

BARBIZON 1775 STATE RD 434 W LONGWOOD FL 32750 (407) 331-5558

MARATHON COMMUNITY THEATRE 10888 OVERSEAS HWY MARATHON FL 33050 (305) 743-6529

BREVARD TALENT GROUP INC 405 PALM SPRINGS BLVD MELBOURNE FL 32937 (407) 773-1355

IMAGE GROUP INC 1433 HIGHLAND AVE MELBOURNE FL 32935 (407) 242-9345

ADA GORDON MODEL DIV 1995 NE 150TH ST MIAMI FL 33181 (305) 940-1311

BARBIZON SCHOOL OF MODELING 782 NW 42ND AVE MIAMI FL 33126 (305) 446-8555

BLACK CULTURAL ARTS COALITION 141 NE 3RD AVE MIAMI FL 33132 (305) 379-6025

COCONUT GROVE TALENT AGENCY 3525 VISTA CT MIAMI FL 33133 (305) 858-3002

INTERNATIONAL MODELS INC 8415 CORAL WAY # 205 MIAMI FL 33155 (305) 266-6331

JOHN CASABLANCAS MODELING CTR 10491 N KENDALL DR MIAMI FL 33176 (305) 279-0101

KENDALL MODELS 12926 SW 133RD CT MIAMI FL 33186 (305) 232-8650

LITTLE KIDDIES PRODUCTION 3971 SW 8TH ST MIAMI FL 33134 (305) 444-8806

MAR BEA TALENT AGENCY 1946 NE 149TH ST MIAMI FL 33181 (305) 949-0615

MODE MODEL & TALENT MANAGEMENT 1110 BRICKELL AVE MIAMI FL 33131 (305) 358-0201

*POMMIER KIDS DIV 81 WASHINGTON AVE MIAMI FL 33139 (305) 672-9344

PROMESA MANAGEMENT 770 CLAUGHTON ISLAND DR MIAMI FL 33131 (305) 372-9696

RUNWAYS FLORIDA MODELS ASSN 9350 S DIXIE HWY MIAMI FL 33156 (305) 670-3003

STARTERS MODEL PRODUCTION CO 15050 NE 20TH AVE MIAMI FL 33181 (305) 940-5010

TALENT SEEKERS CONSULTANTS 15120 SW 69TH CT MIAMI FL 33158 (305) 233-5815

UNITED STARS 999 S BAYSHORE DR MIAMI FL 33131 (305) 374-7137

WORLD PAGEANTS INC 18761 W DIXIE HWY # 284 MIAMI FL 33180 (305) 933-2993

*ACT I MODEL & TALENT AGENCY 1253 WASHINGTON AVE MIAMI BEACH FL 33139 (305) 672-0200

BEAUTY SEARCH MODELS & PAGEANT 420 LINCOLN RD MIAMI BEACH FL 33139 (305) 532-4147

BLACK MODELS NETWORK 1655 DREXEL AVE # 206 MIAMI BEACH FL 33139 (305) 531-2700

*CLICK MODELS MIAMI 161 OCEAN DR MIAMI BEACH FL 33139 (305) 674-9900

DANIEL BATES INTL MANAGEMENT 81 WASHINGTON AVE MIAMI BEACH FL 33139 (305) 538-3900

DIAMOND BULLET CORP 930 WASHINGTON AVE MIAMI BEACH FL 33139 (305) 532-1566

*ELITE MODEL MANAGEMENT MIAMI 1200 COLLINS AVE MIAMI BEACH FL 33139 (305) 674-9500

ELLEN JACOBY CASTING INTL LTD 420 LINCOLN RD MIAMI BEACH FL 33139 (305) 531-5300

FLICK EAST WEST TALENT 161 OCEAN DR MIAMI BEACH FL 33139 (305) 538-4887

*FORD MODELS INC 826 OCEAN DR MIAMI BEACH FL 33139 (305) 534-7200

*GREEN & GREEN 1688 MERIDIAN AVE MIAMI BEACH FL 33139 (305) 532-9880

IMAGE LIFESTYLE TALENT AGENCY 420 LINCOLN RD MIAMI BEACH FL 33139 (305) 531-9096

INTERNATIONAL ARTISTS GROUP 420 LINCOLN RD MIAMI BEACH FL 33139 (305) 538-6100

INTERNATIONAL TALENT CORP 1130 WASHINGTON AVE MIAMI BEACH FL 33139 (305) 531-5700

*L'AGENCE INC 850 OCEAN DR MIAMI BEACH FL 33139 (305) 672-0804

MEN'S BOARD 850 OCEAN DR MIAMI BEACH FL 33139 (305) 531-1610

MIAMI MODELS & TALENT AGENCY 411 WASHINGTON AVE MIAMI BEACH FL 33139 (305) 531-6924

*MICHELE POMMIER MODELS INC 81 WASHINGTON AVE MIAMI BEACH FL 33139 (305) 531-5475

*NEXT MANAGEMENT CO 209 9TH ST MIAMI BEACH FL 33139 (305) 531-5100

*PAGE PARKES MODEL'S REP 660 OCEAN DR MIAMI BEACH FL 33139 (305) 672-4869

PAPER DOLLS 420 LINCOLN RD MIAMI BEACH FL 33139 (305) 255-2407

PLUS MODELS 1400 OCEAN DR MIAMI BEACH FL 33139 (305) 672-9882

RAVEN INTERNATIONAL 1688 MERIDIAN AVE MIAMI BEACH FL 33139 (305) 531-1003

REAL CREATIVE 1253 WASHINGTON AVE MIAMI BEACH FL 33139 (305) 674-1113

RITA'S INTERNATIONAL MODELING 227 13TH ST # 3 MIAMI BEACH FL 33139 (305) 534-3034

SELECT MODELS 817 WASHINGTON AVE MIAMI BEACH FL 33139 (305) 672-5566

STELLAR MODEL & TALENT AGENCY 407 LINCOLN RD MIAMI BEACH FL 33139 (305) 672-2217

WORLD OF KIDS INC 1460 OCEAN DR MIAMI BEACH FL 33139 (305) 672-5437

CHARMETTE CHARM & MODELING INC 500 DEER RUN MIAMI SPRINGS FL 33166 (305) 870-0509

FASHIONCREST FASHION SHOWS 135 WESTWARD DR MIAMI SPRINGS FL 33166 (305) 887-2115

PREMIERE MODEL MANAGEMENT 223 N CSWY NEW SMYRNA BEACH FL 32169 (904) 427-8829

HOLLYWOOD CASTING GROUP 12100 NE 16TH AVE NORTH MIAMI FL 33161 (305) 891-7225

INTERNATIONAL SPORTS AGENCY 1175 NE 125TH ST NORTH MIAMI FL 33161 (305) 895-3388

MODEL & TALENT INTL INC 12100 NE 16TH AVE NORTH MIAMI FL 33161 (305) 891-7003

ARIE KADURI AGENCY INC 16125 NE 18TH AVE NORTH MIAMI BCH FL 33162 (305) 949-3055

BEVERLY HILLS TALENT MGMT 3365 N FEDERAL HWY OAKLAND PARK FL 33306 (954) 565-4994

*CASSANDRA & BAILEY MODELS 513 W COLONIAL DR ORLANDO FL 32804 (407) 843-3215

*CASSANDRA AGENCY-HOSTESS 513 W COLONIAL DR ORLANDO FL 32804 (407) 422-1008

CHILDREN & EXTRAS 513 W COLONIAL DR ORLANDO FL 32804 (407) 422-1008

CREATIVE TALENT AGENCY 4301 VINELAND RD ORLANDO FL 32811 (407) 872-6231

DIMENSIONS III MODELING & TLNT 5205 S ORANGE AVE ORLANDO FL 32809 (407) 851-2575

DIVA MODELS & TALENT 7041 GRAND NATL DR # 1281 ORLANDO FL 32819 (407) 352-3795

EXTRA EXPRESS 2000 UNIVERSAL STUDIOS PLZ ORLANDO FL 32819 (407) 363-0717

HILL MODELING & TALENT AGENCY 5728 MAJOR BLVD ORLANDO FL 32819 (407) 345-0075

MODELSCOUT INC 651 RUGBY ST ORLANDO FL 32804 (407) 420-5888

PHILLIP KARR TALENT AGENCY 5979 VINELAND RD ORLANDO FL 32819 (407) 363-7773

DAVID CRANE AGENCY 505 RIVERSIDE DR ORMOND BEACH FL 32176 (904) 672-1550

IN ANY EVENT 140 S ATLANTIC AVE ORMOND BEACH FL 32176 (904) 676-2223

MICHELE & GROUP MODELING AGCY 305 W GRANADA BLVD ORMOND BEACH FL 32174 (904) 676-1702

JONATHAN ROBINSON THEATRICAL 4610 LIPSCOMB ST NE PALM BAY FL 32905 (407) 727-7727

MICAH'S MODELS 17320 PANAMA CITY BEACH PKY PANAMA CITY BCH FL 32413 (904) 234-0286

BARBIZON SCHOOL OF MODELING 8385 PINES BLVD PEMBROKE PINES FL 33024 (954) 437-7900

IMAGES MODELING AGENCY INC 744 E BURGESS RD PENSACOLA FL 32504 (904) 484-7725

PAZAZZ MODELING & TALENT 14110 PERDIDO KEY DR PENSACOLA FL 32507 (904) 492-2725

FLORIDA TALENT & MODEL MGMT 10707 66TH ST PINELLAS PARK FL 33782 (813) 545-8686

SOUTH FLORIDA MODELS 1650 N FEDERAL HWY POMPANO BEACH FL 33062 (954) 781-0308

MASTERPIECE MODELS 7642 S TAMIAMI TRL SARASOTA FL 34231 (941) 927-8415

SEA STARS TALENT AGENCY INC 1266 1ST ST SARASOTA FL 34236 (941) 955-5341

SUZI'S INTERNATIONAL MODELS 2426 BEE RIDGE RD SARASOTA FL 34239 (941) 922-5339

STEPHANIE GIBBS MODELS & TLNT 1365 S PATRICK DR SATELLITE BEACH FL 32937 (407) 777-9127

JUDITH GINDY TALENT AGENCY 7615 SW 62ND AVE SOUTH MIAMI FL 33143 (305) 666-3470

CENTRAL CASTING STOKES LANDING RD ST AUGUSTINE FL 32095 (904) 824-6533

MAR BEA TALENT AGENCY 24 CATHEDRAL PL ST AUGUSTINE FL 32084 (904) 826-0939

CONTINENTAL THEATRICAL AGENCY 7605 COQUINA WAY ST PETERSBRG BCH FL 33706 (813) 363-7100

*SMARTER IMAGE INC 1344 SE MACARTHUR BLVD STUART FL 34994 (561) 288-1188

TURNABOUT MODELING SCHOOL 584 SE MONTEREY RD STUART FL 34994 (561) 283-1449

KIDS & CO MANAGEMENT 11710 NW 39TH PL SUNRISE FL 33323 (954) 748-9123

*MARSHA DOLL MODELS & TALENT 2131 ORLEANS DRIVE TALLAHASSEE FL 32308 (904) 656-2600

SET FIVE MODELS & TALENT 714 GLENVIEW DR TALLAHASSEE FL 32303 (904) 224-8500

*ALEXA MODEL & TALENT MGMT AGCY 4100 W KENNEDY BLVD # 228 TAMPA FL 33609 (813) 289-8020

BERG TALENT AGENCY 1115 N HIMES AVE TAMPA FL 33607 (813) 877-5533

BOOK & CO 111 E MADISON ST TAMPA FL 33602 (813) 223-6335

*BOOM MODEL & TALENT AGENCY 13012 N. DALEMABRY HWY, STE B TAMPA FL 33607 (813) 264-1373

DESIGNS MODELING & ACTING CTR 4707 E BUSCH BLVD TAMPA FL 33617 (813) 914-0809

*DOTT BURNS TALENT AGENCY 478 SEVERN TAMPA FL 33606 (813) 251-5882

JOHN CASABLANCAS MODELING CTR 5215 W LAUREL ST # 110 TAMPA FL 33607 (813) 289-8564

MODELMANIA INC 3200 HENDERSON BLVD TAMPA FL 33609 (813) 877-2255

ON LOCATION MODELING 1408 N WESTSHORE BLVD TAMPA FL 33607 (813) 289-6356

SUN COAST MODELS TALENT 5915 MEMORIAL HWY TAMPA FL 33615 (813) 884-8841

TRENDS MODEL TALENT INC 2900 E 7TH AVE TAMPA FL 33605 (813) 248-4008

TURNABOUT MODELING SCHOOL 740 BEACHLAND BLVD VERO BEACH FL 32963 (561) 231-4579

FINLEY & ASSOC 1645 PALM BEACH LAKES BLVD # 300 WEST PALM BEACH FL 33401 (561) 478-9930

MODELING RESOURCE CTR 1300 N FLORIDA MANGO RD WEST PALM BEACH FL 33409 (561) 688-1009

SARAH PARKER'S MODEL & TALENT 410 DATURA ST WEST PALM BEACH FL 33401 (561) 686-7201

AZUREE TALENT AGENCY 140 N ORLANDO AVE # 120 WINTER PARK FL 32789 (407) 629-5025

CASABLANCAS MODELING & CAREER 329 S PARK AVE # 200 WINTER PARK FL 32789 (407) 740-6697

HURT-GARVER TALENT & MODELS 400 N NEW YORK AVE WINTER PARK FL 32789 (407) 740-5700

LISA MAILE IMAGE MODELING 999 S ORLANDO AVE WINTER PARK FL 32789 (407) 628-5989

MODEL CAMP INC 2311 FORREST RD WINTER PARK FL 32789 (407) 647-6336

STRICTLY SPEAKING INC 711 EXECUTIVE DR WINTER PARK FL 32789 (407) 645-2111

SUSANNE HALEY TALENT 618 N WYMORE RD WINTER PARK FL 32789 (407) 644-0600

GEORGIA

AGENCY BURNETTE-JLH ENTERPRISE 741 PIEDMONT AVE NE ATLANTA GA 30308 (404) 875-0398

*ARLENE WILSON MODEL MANAGEMENT 887 W MARIETTA ST NW ATLANTA GA 30318 (404) 876-8555

*ATLANTA MODELS & TALENT INC 2970 PEACHTREE RD NW ATLANTA GA 30305 (404) 261-9627

ATLANTA TALENT SEARCH 2873 PINE GROVE TER NE ATLANTA GA 30319 (404) 848-9930

ATLANTA'S YOUNG FACES 6075 ROSWELL RD NE ATLANTA GA 30328 (404) 255-3080

AUSTON'S PROFESSIONAL MODELING 3391 NE PEACHTREE RD # 410 ATLANTA GA 30326 (404) 237-9800

B B BABIES MODELING SCHOOL INC 1776 PEACHTREE ST NW ATLANTA GA 30309 (404) 870-0963

BARBIZON SCHOOL OF MODELING 3340 NE PEACHTREE RD # 120 ATLANTA GA 30326 (404) 261-7332

BELLE'S MODELS & TALENT 643 11TH ST NW ATLANTA GA 30318 (404) 607-7277

BOHANNON MODELING AGENCY 4820 OLD NATL HWY ATLANTA GA 30337 (404) 209-0909

CASTING CONNECTION INC 300 W PEACHTREE ST NW ATLANTA GA 30308 (404) 221-0400

CHADZ MODEL MGMT 3108 PIEDMONT RD NE ATLANTA GA 30305 (404) 261-4969

*CHEZ GROUP 1776 PEACHTREE RD NW ATLANTA GA 30309 (404) 873-1215

*CLICK MODEL MIA 2970 PEACHTREE RD NW ATLANTA GA 30305 (404) 233-2029

CREWS 2004 ROCKLEDGE RD NE ATLANTA GA 30324 (404) 876-6880

*ELITE MODEL MANAGEMENT CORP 181 14TH ST NE ATLANTA GA 30309 (404) 872-7444

ELLIS-CROSS ASSOC INC 1422 W PEACHTREE ST NW ATLANTA GA 30309 (404) 874-1709

GENESIS MODELS & TALENT INC 1465 NORTHSIDE DR NW ATLANTA GA 30318 (404) 350-9212

GLYN KENNEDY MODEL & TALENT 659 NE PEACHTREE ST # 1500 ATLANTA GA 30308 (404) 892-5500

HOUGHTON AGENCY INC 2810 NEW SPRING RD NW ATLANTA GA 30339 (770) 433-0301

JOHN CASABLANCAS MODEL & TLNT 6255 NE BARFIELD RD # 165 ATLANTA GA 30328 (404) 705-9494

JOHN F TEMPLETON MODEL & TLNT 73 WADDELL ST NE ATLANTA GA 30307 (404) 688-4101

JUDY VENN & ASSOC INC 13 FORREST PL NE ATLANTA GA 30328 (770) 579-2888

KIDDIN' AROUND MODELS & TALENT 1479 SPRING ST NW ATLANTA GA 30309 (404) 872-8582

*L'AGENCE MODELS 5901 NE PEACHTREE DUN RD # 60 ATLANTA GA 30328 (770) 396-9015

LILLIE DUMAS MODEL AGENCY 5495 OLD NATL HWY ATLANTA GA 30349 (404) 305-9871

MADISON AGENCY 2814 NW NEW SPRING RD # 103 ATLANTA GA 30339 (770) 432-2115

*MICHELE POMMIER ATLANTA 1 NW BALTIMORE PL # 360 ATLANTA GA 30308 (404) 815-5888

MISS GEORGIA/FLORIDA PAGEANT 3391 NE PEACHTREE RD # 410 ATLANTA GA 30326 (404) 233-9300

MODELS BY LAME' 1776 PEACHTREE ST NW ATLANTA GA 30309 (404) 815-2992

PEOPLE STORE INC 2004 ROCKLEDGE RD NE ATLANTA GA 30324 (404) 874-6448

POPE MODELING CONSULTANT 3060 N PHARR CT NW ATLANTA GA 30305 (404) 261-0736

REAL PEOPLE 1479 SPRING ST NW ATLANTA GA 30309 (404) 872-4007

*SERINDIPITY MODELS INTL INC 550 NE PHARR RD # 220 ATLANTA GA 30305 (404) 237-4040

TALENT PARTNERS 4840 ROSWELL RD NE ATLANTA GA 30342 (404) 303-8030

TED BORDEN & ASSOC 2434 ADINA DR NE ATLANTA GA 30324 (404) 266-0664

TMA TALENTS 1702 DUNWOODY PL NE ATLANTA GA 30324 (404) 231-1778

WILLIAM REYNOLDS AGENCY 1932 N DRUID HILLS RD # 100 ATLANTA GA 30319 (404) 636-1974

ALL AMERICAN MODELING 3830 WASHINGTON RD # 24 AUGUSTA GA 30907 (706) 860-5425

DYSART MODELING TALENT & CSTNG 55 TIBURON TRAIL AUGUSTA GA 30907 (706) 868-7221

TUNNEL VISION 3300 BUCKEYE RD CHAMBLEE GA 30341 (770) 451-8266

EMB 3729 MAIN ST COLLEGE PARK GA 30337 (404) 209-1002

BABES 4337 VICTORY DR COLUMBUS GA 31903 (706) 687-2553

MABLE BAILEY FASHION COLLEGE 3121 CROSS COUNTRY HL COLUMBUS GA 31906 (706) 563-0606

MADEMOISELLE MODELING AGENCY 2901 UNIVERSITY AVE COLUMBUS GA 31907 (706) 561-9449

ALIEN BOOKING 623 WEBSTER DR DECATUR GA 30033 (404) 320-9191

BURNS AGENCY INC 602 HAMMETT DR DECATUR GA 30032 (404) 299-8114

ONE G BOOKING AGENCY 4488 DORSET DR DECATUR GA 30035 (770) 981-3952

TARA MODELING ACADEMY 650 MORROW INDUSTRIAL BLVD JONESBORO GA 30236 (770) 968-7700

LEE MODEL & TALENT AGENCY PO BOX 2313 KENNESAW GA 30144 (770) 966-9988

MODELING IMAGES 2106 CHATOU PL KENNESAW GA 30152 (770) 565-4581

SNIKKERS AMI 2749 ELMHURST BLVD KENNESAW GA 30152 (770) 428-5484

EXCLAMATIONS MODEL/TALENT AGCY 670 HILLCREST RD NW LILBURN GA 30247 (770) 925-8888

TOSHA REID ENTERPRISES 548 BROADWAY MACON GA 31201 (912) 755-1070

ALTANTA BEST TALENT 1850 PKY PL MARIETTA GA 30067 (770) 424-5158

BABES 'N BEAUS 4757 CANTON RD MARIETTA GA 30066 (770) 928-5832

MODELING SHOP 401 ATLANTA ST MARIETTA GA 30060 (770) 424-6077

SHOWSTOPPERS PAGENT & TALENT HIGHWAY 41 RINGGOLD GA 30736 (706) 891-7324

LORREN & MACY'S MODELING 405 BROAD ST # A ROME GA 30161 (706) 235-1175

*MILLIE LEWIS OF SAVANNAH 7011 HODGSON MEMORIAL DR SAVANNAH GA 31406 (912) 354-9525

TALENT SOURCE 107 E HALL ST SAVANNAH GA 31401 (912) 232-9390

MISS BLACK GEORGIA PAGEANTS 5368 FIELDGREEN DR STONE MOUNTAIN GA 30088 (770) 498-0081

A J CARRINGTON ACTING & MDLNG 4303 LAVISTA RD TUCKER GA 30084 (770) 270-9303

COLOURS OF THE WORLD MODELS 2533 N ASHLEY ST VALDOSTA GA 31602 (912) 244-8929

LIZ UNIQUE SCHOOL OF MODELING 502 N PATTERSON ST VALDOSTA GA 31601 (912) 245-9934

SYLVIA'S MODELS & TALENT AGCY 1011 WILLIAMS ST VALDOSTA GA 31601 (912) 244-9275

Hawaii

MODEL'S INC 98 HEKAHA ST # 223A AIEA HI 96701 (808) 484-1257

KANIU KINIMAKA MODEL & TALENT 69 RAILROAD AVE HILO HI 96720 (808) 961-0031

ABEL MODEL & TALENT AGENCY 680 ALA MOANA BLVD # 306 HONOLULU HI 96813 (808) 536-4122

ACE OF HEARTS MODELS & TALENT 801 ALA NIOI PL # 1102 HONOLULU HI 96818 (808) 839-6934

ADR MODEL & TALENT AGENCY PO BOX 61969 HONOLULU HI 96839 (808) 524-4777

AGENCE POWERS 1314 S KING ST # 504 HONOLULU HI 96814 (808) 596-8165

FIRST MODEL MANAGEMENT INC 1335 RIVER ST # 211 HONOLULU HI 96817 (808) 599-5515

INTERNATIONAL TALENT AGENCY 1111 BISHOP ST HONOLULU HI 96813 (808) 533-1669

JOHN ROBERT POWERS MODELING 1314 S KING ST # 504 HONOLULU HI 96814 (808) 596-2800

KATHY MULLER TALENT & MODELING 619 KAPAHULU AVE HONOLULU HI 96815 (808) 737-7917

KOTOMORI AGENCY 1018 HOAWA LN HONOLULU HI 96826 (808) 955-6511

MEWS 845 MISSION LN HONOLULU HI 96813 (808) 524-2022

OMNIQUE LIMITED 1750 KALAKAUA AVE # 103 HONOLULU HI 96826 (808) 944-3382

SOHBI'S TALENT AGENCY 1750 KALAKAUA AVE # 204B HONOLULU HI 96826 (808) 946-6614

SUSAN PAGE MODELING & TALENT 1441 KAPIOLANI BLVD # 1206 HONOLULU HI 96814 (808) 955-2271

VOGUE INTERNATIONAL MODELING 2153 N KING ST # 323A HONOLULU HI 96819 (808) 842-0881

ENCORE TALENT 77 AINANANI ST KAILUA KONA HI 96740 (808) 326-1636

CHAMELEON TALENT AGENCY 590 LIPOA PKY KIHEI HI 96753 (808) 875-2511

BEAUTIFUL BABIES MODELING WAIMANALO HI 96795 (808) 259-7236

CIA CENTRAL ISLAND AGENCY 41 LAUMILO ST WAIMANALO HI 96795 (808) 259-7914

Iowa

ADA GAFFNEY SHAFF CHARM SCHOOL 2828 18TH ST # 1 BETTENDORF IA 52722 (319) 359-6144

AVANT MODELS & TALENT 7600 UNIVERSITY AVE DES MOINES IA 50325 (515) 255-0297

COPELAND CREATIVE TALENT 4140 GRAND AVE # A DES MOINES IA 50312 (515) 271-5970

MODEL CONSULTANTS 2625 SE 18TH ST DES MOINES IA 50320 (515) 244-5500

TALENT/IOWA 6545 SE BLOOMFIELD RD DES MOINES IA 50320 (515) 285-8907

WINNING COMBINATIONS 5714 MCKINLEY AVE DES MOINES IA 50321 (515) 287-2100

DAVID JOHN FASHION THEATRE 109 1ST ST SE MASON CITY IA 50401 (515) 423-9483

AMERICAN ETHNIC MODEL AGENCY 326 N WALNUT ST MONTICELLO IA 52310 (319) 395-7772

CORRINE SHOVER SCHOOLS 326 N WALNUT ST MONTICELLO IA 52310 (319) 465-5507

MIRAGE INTERNATIONAL MODELING 4920 CEDAR DR WEST DES MOINES IA 50266 (515) 225-2221

IDAHO

BLANCHE B EVANS SCHOOL & AGCY 404 S 8TH ST BOISE ID 83702 (208) 344-5380

JAN-JON 290 BOBWHITE CT # 120 BOISE ID 83706 (208) 387-4900

METCALF'S MODELING & TALENT 1851 CENTURY WAY # 3 BOISE ID 83709 (208) 378-8777

NATIONAL SCOUTING REPORT 1020 MAIN ST # 440 BOISE ID 83702 (208) 343-3438

COEUR D ALENE MODELING AGENCY PO BOX 1002 COEUR D ALENE ID 83816 (208) 664-5278

UNITED MODELS 106 N WOODRUFF AVE IDAHO FALLS ID 83401 (208) 529-3771

TALENT POOL 326 17TH AVE LEWISTON ID 83501 (208) 743-4352

LAMEE AGENCY 3764 SUGAR CREEK DR MERIDIAN ID 83642 (208) 888-7319

ILLINOIS

FOX VALLEY THEATRES 4001 FOX VALLEY CTR AURORA IL 60504 (630) 851-7280

LEA CONSULTING 1345 CARLISLE DR BARRINGTON IL 60010 (847) 382-6640

JUDY VENN & ASSOC INC 1448 HOLBROOK LN BATAVIA IL 60510 (630) 879-9970

AUDITION DIVISION LTD 1084 INDUSTRIAL DR BENSENVILLE IL 60106 (630) 766-6100

THIRD STONE BOOKING 41 E UNIVERSITY AVE CHAMPAIGN IL 61820 (217) 355-1950

ACTOR'S CONNECTION 676 N LA SALLE # 418 CHICAGO IL 60610 (312) 464-3230

AL DVORIN AGENCY 2701 W HOWARD ST CHICAGO IL 60645 (773) 743-8500

ALL ABOUT MODELS TALENT 435 N LA SALLE ST # 204 CHICAGO IL 60610 (312) 527-4500

AMBASSADOR TALENT BOOKING AGCY 333 N MICHIGAN AVE CHICAGO IL 60601 (312) 641-3491

ARIA MODEL & TALENT MGMT LTD 1017 W WASHINGTON BLVD CHICAGO IL 60607 (312) 243-9400

*ARLENE WILSON MODEL & TALENT 430 W ERIE ST # 210 CHICAGO IL 60610 (312) 573-0200

BARBIZON MODELING AGENCY 541 N FAIRBANKS CT CHICAGO IL 60611 (312) 329-9405

BARBIZON SCHOOL OF MODELING 541 N FAIRBANKS CT CHICAGO IL 60611 (312) 321-6200

BEST FACES OF CHICAGO 1152 N LA SALLE DR CHICAGO IL 60610 (312) 944-3009

BILL'S MODELING STUDIO 7447 S SHORE DR CHICAGO IL 60649 (773) 731-4220

CARLA WALCH MODELING CONSLNTS 2001 N ELSTON AVE CHICAGO IL 60614 (773) 489-4590

CHICAGO FASHION ASSOC 202 S STATE ST CHICAGO IL 60604 (312) 461-0725

CHICAGO MODEL 4722 N BEACON ST CHICAGO IL 60640 (773) 728-7545

CHICAGO MODEL & TALENT MGMT 435 N LA SALLE DR # 100 CHICAGO IL 60610 (312) 527-2977

CHICAGO TALENT ENTERPRISES INC 1436 W SUMMERDALE AVE CHICAGO IL 60640 (773) 728-3800

DAVID & LEE MODEL MANAGEMENT 70 W HUBBARD ST CHICAGO IL 60610 (312) 661-0500

*ELITE MODEL MANAGEMENT CORP 212 W SUPERIOR ST # 406 CHICAGO IL 60610 (312) 943-3226

ETA CREATIVE ARTS FOUNDATION 7558 S CHICAGO AVE CHICAGO IL 60619 (773) 752-3955

GROUP 5757 N SHERIDAN RD CHICAGO IL 60660 (773) 769-4437

HARRISE DAVIDSON & ASSOC INC 65 E WACKER PL CHICAGO IL 60601 (312) 782-4480

INTERLINGUA WORLDWIDE 333 N MICHIGAN AVE # 3200 CHICAGO IL 60601 (312) 782-8123

INTRIGUE TALENT AGENCY 6151 N WINTHROP AVE CHICAGO IL 60660 (773) 761-1032

JANE ALDERMAN CASTING 2105 N SOUTHPORT AVE CHICAGO IL 60614 (773) 549-6464

JEFFERSON & ASSOC 1050 N STATE ST CHICAGO IL 60610 (312) 337-1930

JOHN CASABLANCAS STUDIOS 435 N LA SALLE DR CHICAGO IL 60610 (312) 329-2000

JOHN ROBERT POWERS MODELING 27 E MONROE ST # 200 CHICAGO IL 60603 (312) 726-1404

JOUSTING KNIGHTS & STEEDS 3708 N HERMITAGE AVE CHICAGO IL 60613 (773) 404-4376

KIDS R PEOPLE 2 1020 S WABASH AVE CHICAGO IL 60605 (312) 408-1900

LILY'S TALENT AGENCY INC 5962 N ELSTON AVE CHICAGO IL 60646 (773) 792-1160

M L INTL MODELING INC 162 N FRANKLIN ST CHICAGO IL 60606 (312) 849-9190

MC DONALD MODEL MANAGEMENT 3214 N RAVENSWOOD AVE CHICAGO IL 60657 (773) 525-3863

MODELS WORKSHOP STUDIO 118 W KINZIE ST CHICAGO IL 60610 (312) 527-2807

MONTEREY INTERNATIONAL 200 W SUPERIOR ST CHICAGO IL 60610 (312) 640-7500

NATIONAL TALENT ASSOC 6326 N LINCOLN AVE CHICAGO IL 60659 (773) 539-8575

NORTH SHORE TALENT INC 152 W HURON ST CHICAGO IL 60610 (847) 816-1811

NORTH SHORE THEATER CO 525 W HAWTHORNE PL CHICAGO IL 60657 (773) 296-2196

PALM GROUP LTD 345 N CANAL ST CHICAGO IL 60606 (312) 382-5368

PARTIMERS INC 69 W WASHINGTON ST CHICAGO IL 60602 (312) 464-2039

SALAZAR & NAVAS TALENT AGENCY 367 W CHICAGO AVE CHICAGO IL 60610 (312) 751-3419

SHIRLEY HAMILTON INC 333 E ONTARIO ST CHICAGO IL 60611 (312) 787-4700

STEVEN IVCICH STUDIO 1836 W NORTH AVE CHICAGO IL 60622 (773) 235-9131

STEWART TALENT AGENCY 212 W SUPERIOR ST CHICAGO IL 60610 (312) 943-3131

*SUSANNE JOHNSON TALENT AGENCY 108 W OAK ST CHICAGO IL 60610 (312) 943-8315

SWOPES MODELING & TALENT NTWRK 185 N WABASH AVE CHICAGO IL 60601 (312) 236-2378

TALENT GROUP 4637 N MAGNOLIA AVE CHICAGO IL 60640 (773) 561-8814

*TLW MODELING & PROMOTIONS 101 W GRAND AVE CHICAGO IL 60610 (312) 645-0880

VOICES UNLIMITED 680 N LAKE SHORE DR CHICAGO IL 60611 (312) 642-3262

AMBIANCE CHICAGO INC 316 DIXIE HWY CHICAGO HEIGHTS IL 60411 (708) 754-7272

DRAMA GROUP 330 202ND ST CHICAGO HEIGHTS IL 60411 (708) 755-3444

BIANCHI MODELING AGENCY 1626 DURHAM CT CRYSTAL LAKE IL 60014 (815) 477-1280

STEWART'S NORTHWEST TALENT 4227 CONNECTICUT TRL CRYSTAL LAKE IL 60012 (815) 455-6311

TNT PRODUCTIONS INC 41 N VERMILION ST DANVILLE IL 61832 (217) 446-9120

LAURA VIA INC 1052 HINSWOOD DR DARIEN IL 60561 (630) 241-1010

CASTING CALL INC 430 WESTERN ST HOFFMAN ESTATES IL 60194 (847) 885-7810

APPEARANCE PLUS 633 S LA GRANGE RD LA GRANGE IL 60525 (708) 246-9140

NORTH SHORE TALENT INC 454 PETERSON RD LIBERTYVILLE IL 60048 (847) 816-1811

MARKETING UNLIMITED MODELING 1921 5TH AVE MOLINE IL 61265 (309) 762-6893

SHAWNEE STUDIOS 102 W MAIN ST MT OLIVE IL 62069 (217) 999-2522

RICHARD MARRIOTT & ASSOC 1727 W CRYSTAL LN MT PROSPECT IL 60056 (847) 593-5309

HOWARD W SCHULTZ THEATRICAL 241 GOLF MILL CTR NILES IL 60714 (847) 390-0600

ALL ABOUT MODELS TALENT 555 SKOKIE BLVD NORTHBROOK IL 60062 (847) 509-1555

KIDSTAGE PRODUCTIONS 2654 ILLINOIS RD NORTHBROOK IL 60062 (847) 559-8790

MODEL IMAGE CTR INC 1512 SHERMER RD NORTHBROOK IL 60062 (312) 348-9349

ANNE O'BRIANT AGENCY 11819 CHISHOLM TRL ORLAND PARK IL 60462 (708) 460-3677

ARNOLD & BROWN 6707 N SHERIDAN RD PEORIA IL 61614 (309) 691-7104

GLAMOUR GIRL CHARM SCHOOL 2601 N MISSION RD PEORIA IL 61604 (309) 682-4266

NEW STAR DISCOVERY 2426 S ALPINE RD ROCKFORD IL 61108 (815) 227-1070

ELEGANT MODEL INC 6132 BYRON ST ROSEMONT IL 60018 (847) 825-3685

BARBIZON SCHOOL OF MODELING 1051 PERIMETER DR SCHAUMBURG IL 60173 (847) 240-4200

ROYAL MODEL MANAGEMENT 1051 PERIMETER DR SCHAUMBURG IL 60173 (847) 240-4215

DELLA M GALLO INDEPENDENT THTR 5225 TOUHY AVE SKOKIE IL 60077 (847) 675-8232

CHICAGO MODEL PRODUCTION 17 22ND ST VILLA PARK IL 60181 (630) 530-5600

SGA PRODUCTIONS STAGING 3 TIMBER DR WARRENVILLE IL 60555 (630) 393-3432

CHICAGO IMAGES MODELING AGENCY 925 N MILWAUKEE AVE WHEELING IL 60090 (847) 465-8881

CLAIRE MODEL & TALENT WHEELING IL 60090 (847) 459-4242

GENEVA INTERNATIONAL CORP 29 E HINTZ RD WHEELING IL 60090 (847) 520-9970

INDIANA

HELEN WELLS INC 11711 N MERIDIAN ST CARMEL IN 46032 (317) 843-5363

SUPER MODELS INTL 14420 CHERRY TREE RD CARMEL IN 46033 (317) 846-4321

FINISHING TOUCH MODELING AGCY 2500 HARMONY WAY EVANSVILLE IN 47720 (812) 422-5064

JOYCE'S STARS OF TOMORROW 4004 E MORGAN AVE # 202 EVANSVILLE IN 47715 (812) 473-0466

CHARMAINE SCHOOL & MODEL AGCY 3538 STELLHORN RD FORT WAYNE IN 46815 (219) 485-8421

CORRAINE TALENT AGENCY INC 2711 N WELLS ST FORT WAYNE IN 46808 (219) 471-4299

ACT I MODEL & TALENT AGENCY 6100 N KEYSTONE AVE # 105 INDIANAPOLIS IN 46220 (317) 255-3100

EVE'S AGENCY 2625 N MERIDIAN ST # 204 INDIANAPOLIS IN 46208 (317) 924-3787

KRISTIE OF CHICAGO INC 9000 KEYSTONE XING # 230 INDIANAPOLIS IN 46240 (317) 846-9656

MODEL MAKERS INC 10 W MARKET ST INDIANAPOLIS IN 46204 (317) 464-5215

ONLY IN AMERICA MODELING 2721 E 56TH ST INDIANAPOLIS IN 46220 (317) 251-7021

UNION STREET MODELING & TALENT 1 VIRGINIA AVE # 101 INDIANAPOLIS IN 46204 (317) 261-9235

AAA MODELING & TALENT AGENCY 736 10TH PL MISHAWAKA IN 46544 219 2557275

BEAUTY & THE BEST INC 249 BARBERRY LN E VALPARAISO IN 46383 (219) 477-6603

KANSAS

AGENCY MODELS & TALENT 3025 MERRIAM LN KANSAS CITY KS 66106 (913) 362-8382

AGENCY MODELS & TALENT 116 GREYSTONE AVE KANSAS CITY KS 66103 (913) 342-8382

CAREER IMAGES MODEL & TALENT 8519 LATHROP AVE KANSAS CITY KS 66109 (913) 334-2200

CASTING PLACE 4024 STATE LINE RD KANSAS CITY KS 66103 (913) 831-0060

TALENT SEARCH 4601 STATE AVE KANSAS CITY KS 66102 (913) 596-1701

OZARK TALENT 718 SCHWARZ RD LAWRENCE KS 66049 (913) 841-2800

AD-MIX ADVERTISING & MARKETING 2108 W 75TH ST SHAWNEE MISSION KS 66208 (913) 831-9953

HOFFMAN INTERNATIONAL 6705 W 91ST ST SHAWNEE MISSION KS 66212 (913) 642-9294

A TOUCH OF CLASS MODELING SCHL 2719 S CRESTLINE CT WICHITA KS 67215 (316) 721-5599

EBLEUR ELDER IMAGE & CAREER 7701 E KELLOGG DR WICHITA KS 67207 (316) 685-0127

FOCUS MODEL MANAGEMENT 155 N MARKET ST WICHITA KS 67202 (316) 264-3100

GAIL SENN MODELS & PROPS 2300 E DOUGLAS AVE WICHITA KS 67214 (316) 262-8338

GREGORY AGENCY PO BOX 2825 WICHITA KS 67201 (316) 687-5666

J W PRODUCTIONS 2414 N WOODLAWN ST WICHITA KS 67220 (316) 686-5336

J W PRODUCTIONS 550 N 159TH ST E WICHITA KS 67230 (316) 733-9141

KAN TALENT 3915 S SENECA ST WICHITA KS 67217 (316) 522-4599

KINGDOM TALENT 2629 N CHARLES ST WICHITA KS 67204 (316) 838-0030

MODEL'S & IMAGES 1619 N ROCK RD WICHITA KS 67206 (316) 634-2777

RIVER CITY PERFORMING ARTS 3222 E 2ND ST N WICHITA KS 67208 (316) 688-0427

GLAMOUR GIRL MODELING & TNNG 1013 MAIN ST WINFIELD KS 67156 (316) 221-0374

KENTUCKY

ALIX ADAMS SCHOOL-AGENCY 9813 MERIONETH DR JEFFERSONTOWN KY 40299 (502) 266-6990

IMAGES MODEL AGENCY 163 E REYNOLDS RD LEXINGTON KY 40517 (606) 273-2301

VOGUE OF LEXINGTON 1300 NEW CIR RD NE LEXINGTON KY 40505 (606) 254-4582

COSMO MODEL & TALENT 7410 LA GRANGE RD # 204 LOUISVILLE KY 40222 (502) 425-8000

MJK MODELS 414 BAXTER AVE LOUISVILLE KY 40204 (502) 585-4152

PULSE MODEL MANAGEMENT 10410 BLUEGRASS PKY LOUISVILLE KY 40299 (502) 499-5658

STUDIO ELITE INC 11904 PRESTON HWY LOUISVILLE KY 40229 (502) 957-6555

TALENT GROUP 1813 TYLER LN LOUISVILLE KY 40205 (502) 459-3397

TALENT OF KENTUCKY 10410 BLUEGRASS PKY LOUISVILLE KY 40299 (502) 499-5658

VOGUE MODELS INC 2027 FRANKFORT AVE ST MATTHEWS KY 40206 (502) 897-0089

LOUISIANA

DOLLY DEAN MODELING 3617 S SHERWOOD FOREST BLVD BATON ROUGE LA 70816 (504) 292-2424

MODEL & TALENT MANGM 3617 S SHERWOOD FOREST BLVD BATON ROUGE LA 70816 (504) 295-3999

ABOUTFACES MODELING & TALENT 100 E VERMILION ST LAFAYETTE LA 70501 (318) 235-3223

GLAMOUR MODELING AGENCY PO BOX 1526 MERAUX LA 70075 (504) 279-7313

JOHN CASABLANCA'S MODELING 1 GALLERIA BLVD # 825 METAIRIE LA 70001 (504) 831-8000

MTP 1 GALLERIA BLVD # 825 METAIRIE LA 70001 (504) 831-8118

POETRY IN MOTION MODELING 3445 N CSWY BLVD METAIRIE LA 70002 (504) 830-4708

VICTOR'S INTERNATN'L MODEL 3841 VETERANS MEML BLVD # 201 METAIRIE LA 70002 (504) 885-3841

AGENCI' DIRECT MODELING 606 HOMER RD MINDEN LA 71055 (318) 371-0502

ABOUT FACES MODELING & TALENT 201 ST CHARLES AVE # 25 NEW ORLEANS LA 70170 (504) 522-3030

DEL CORRAL MODEL & TALENT 101 W ROBERT LEE BLVD # 205 NEW ORLEANS LA 70124 (504) 288-8963

FAME MODELING & TALENT 1725 CARONDELET ST NEW ORLEANS LA 70130 (504) 522-2001

MODEL MASTERS INC 4346 VAN AVE NEW ORLEANS LA 70122 (504) 288-3315

NEW ORLEANS MODEL & TALENT INC 1347 MAGAZINE ST NEW ORLEANS LA 70130 (504) 525-0100

MICHAEL TURNEY AGENCY 1031 WILKINSON ST SHREVEPORT LA 71104 (318) 221-2628

OMA'S MODELING AGENCY INC 2924 KNIGHT ST # 402 SHREVEPORT LA 71105 (318) 861-2075

MASSACHUSETTS

LA FEMMINA MODELING AGENCY 862 BROCKTON AVE ABINGTON MA 02351 (617) 857-1011

BARBIZON SCHOOL OF MODELING 607 BOYLSTON ST BOSTON MA 02116 (617) 266-6980

CAMEO KIDS MODEL & TALENT AGCY 437 BOYLSTON ST BOSTON MA 02116 (617) 536-6005

CHUTE AGENCY 115 NEWBURY ST BOSTON MA 02116 (617) 262-2626

COPLEY 7 MODELS & TALENT PO BOX 535 BOSTON MA 02117 (617) 267-4444

DYNASTY KIDS 207 NEWBURY ST BOSTON MA 02116 (617) 536-8826

DYNASTY MODELS & TALENT AGENCY 207 NEWBURY ST BOSTON MA 02116 (617) 536-7900

*FORD MODEL MANAGEMENT 297 NEWBURY ST BOSTON MA 02115 (617) 266-6939

IMAGE MAKERS CO 210 LINCOLN ST # 210 BOSTON MA 02111 (617) 482-3622

INTERNATIONAL MODELING AGENCY 25 HUNTINGTON AVE BOSTON MA 02116 (617) 266-5221

JAG MODEL CONSULTANTS 665 BOYLSTON ST BOSTON MA 02116 (617) 424-1124

MAGGIE INC 35 NEWBURY ST BOSTON MA 02116 (617) 536-2639

MODEL CLUB 229 BERKELEY ST BOSTON MA 02116 (617) 247-9020

MODEL CO 224 CLARENDON ST BOSTON MA 02116 (617) 450-9500

MODEL'S GROUP 374 CONGRESS ST BOSTON MA 02210 (617) 426-4711

MODELING CAREER CONCEPTS 297 NEWBURY ST BOSTON MA 02115 (617) 262-9300

MODELS INC 218 NEWBURY ST BOSTON MA 02116 (617) 437-6212

TALENT MANAGEMENT 25 HUNTINGTON AVE BOSTON MA 02116 (617) 424-9577

VIVA INTERNATIONAL MODELING 25 HUNTINGTON AVE # 420 BOSTON MA 02116 (617) 266-0880

WORKSHOP FOR TV MODELING 437 BOYLSTON ST BOSTON MA 02116 (617) 262-1452

LORETTA DAVIS PROMOTIONAL 7 CRESTWOOD DR FRAMINGHAM MA 01701 (508) 872-5919

SPOTLIGHT TALENT CTR & PRMTNS 492 WESTFIELD RD HOLYOKE MA 01040 (413) 532-9772

LA FEMMINA SCHOOL OF MODELING 46 PEARL RD HYANNIS MA 02601 (508) 778-1557

HOT SHOTS MODELING CAREER SCHL 103 CENTRAL ST LOWELL MA 01852 (508) 452-7164

CINDERELLA MODELING AGENCY 65 CLINTON ST MALDEN MA 02148 (617) 324-7590

PRO TEAM THE MODELS & PRMTNS 21 PLEASANT ST NEWBURYPORT MA 01950 (508) 465-9270

MODEL & TALENT MANAGEMENT 1 GATEWAY CTR NEWTON MA 02158 (617) 969-3555

DON GIOVANNI CONSULTING MGMT 1 N PINE ST SALEM MA 01970 (508) 741-1169

BOSTON AGENCY FOR CHILDREN 380 BROADWAY SOMERVILLE MA 02145 (617) 666-0900

PRESTIGE PROMOTIONS 600 W CUMMINGS PARK WOBURN MA 01801 (617) 935-5529

JOHN ROBERT POWERS MODELING 390 MAIN ST # 740 WORCESTER MA 01608 (508) 753-6343

NEW YORK MODEL MANAGEMENT 381 MAIN ST WORCESTER MA 01608 (508) 792-3330

MARYLAND

3 WEST CASTING INC 3 W 23RD ST BALTIMORE MD 21218 (410) 366-7727

BELA NOVA MODEL MANAGEMENT 206 N LIBERTY ST # 3 BALTIMORE MD 21201 (410) 752-6682

CENTRAL CASTING 2229 N CHARLES ST BALTIMORE MD 21218 (410) 889-3274

CHRIS BARRY TALENT CONSULTANT 205 E JOPPA RD BALTIMORE MD 21286 (410) 321-1611

JOHN CASABLANCAS MODELING CTR 7801 YORK RD # 303 BALTIMORE MD 21204 (410) 821-6966

MODEL MANAGEMENT AGENCY INC 7801 YORK RD # 303 BALTIMORE MD 21204 (410) 821-6661

TAYLOR ROYALL CASTING 2308 SO RD BALTIMORE MD 21209 (410) 466-5959

TRAVIS WINKEY MODELING STUDIO 2515 LIBERTY HEIGHTS AVE BALTIMORE MD 21215 (410) 225-7755

LES ANGES TALENT MANAGEMENT 10303 45TH PL BELTSVILLE MD 20705 (301) 937-2527

AWARD AGENCE 7801 NORFOLK AVE # 115 BETHESDA MD 20814 (301) 907-9707

ALL AMERICAN POSTER MODELS 10022 HILLGREEN CIR COCKYSVL HNT VLY MD 21030 (410) 667-4354

BELA MODEL MANAGEMENT 588 BELMAWR PL MILLERSVILLE MD 21108 (410) 987-4336

AQUARIUS MODELS INC 11615 COASTAL HWY # A OCEAN CITY MD 21842 (410) 524-0893

LINDA TOWNSEND MANAGEMENT 1611 BIRCHWOOD DR OXON HILL MD 20745 (301) 567-0531

ANNAPOLIS MODELING AGENCY 130 MANNS RD SEVERNA PARK MD 21146 (410) 647-1200

DAY & NIGHT PRODUCTIONS 3001 GRANITE RD # 2 WOODSTOCK MD 21163 (410) 521-6416

Maine

MID MAINE MODELS & TALENT WINTHROP RD BELGRADE ME 04917 (207) 495-2143

SILHOUETTES MODELING AGENCY 4 CITY CTR PORTLAND ME 04101 (207) 772-1811

PORTLAND MODELS GROUP & TALENT 7 OAK HILL TER SCARBOROUGH ME 04074 (207) 885-5993

Michigan

ABBEY'S PEOPLE 2309 COLUMBIA AVE W BATTLE CREEK MI 49015 (616) 965-8285

TA-DAH PRODUCTIONS 2737 W 12 MILE RD BERKLEY MI 48072 (810) 548-2324

PRODUCTIONS PLUS 30600 TELEGRAPH RD # 2156 BINGHAM FARMS MI 48025 (810) 644-5566

SUCCESS MODELING & TALENT AGCY 101 BROOKSIDE LN BRIGHTON MI 48116 (810) 220-5902

ADVANTAGE 4321 BLUEBIRD ST COMMERCE TWP MI 48382 (810) 363-5500

UNITED TALENT AGENCY 1421 BIRCH CREST ST DEARBORN MI 48124 (810) 414-7177

MODELS UNLIMITED 18437 ROSELAWN ST DETROIT MI 48221 (313) 345-1331

PAMELA PERFILI-USC AGENCY 29441 MEADOW RDG S FARMINGTON MI 48334 (810) 474-9567

STARLITE STAGE PROD   31300 NORTHWESTERN HWY FARMINGTON HILLS MI 48334 (810) 737-9880

ARRAND MODELING SCHOOL & AGCY 13344 WENWOOD DR FENTON MI 48430 (810) 629-7161

AVANTE SCHOOL OF MODELING G3426 MILLER RD # C100 FLINT MI 48507 (810) 732-2233

TALENT SHOP 30100 TELEGRAPH RD # 116 FRANKLIN MI 48025 (810) 644-4877

PASTICHE MODELS & TALENT INC 1514 WEALTHY ST SE GRAND RAPIDS MI 49506 (616) 451-2181

UNIQUE MODELS & TALENT 4485 PLAINFIELD AVE NE GRAND RAPIDS MI 49505 (616) 364-0959

CLASS MODELING TALENT AGENCY 1625 HASLETT RD HASLETT MI 48840 (517) 339-2777

MADELINE'S MODELING AGENCY 4613 W MAIN ST KALAMAZOO MI 49006 (616) 344-0755

I GROUP MODEL TALENT MGMT 28880 SOUTHFIELD RD LATHRUP VILLAGE MI 48076 (810) 552-8842

PROMOTIONAL UNITED MODELING 29200 VASSAR ST LIVONIA MI 48152 (810) 474-6630

MODEL & TALENT MANAGEMENT 44450 PINETREE DR PLYMOUTH MI 48170 (313) 455-0801

AMERICAN MODELS GUILD 3089 YORK RD ROCHESTER HILLS MI 48309 (810) 853-5400

STAR PROJECTIONS 11151 JONATHAN LN ROMEO MI 48065 (810) 752-7464

UNITED TALENT AGENCY BEAUTY 1332 S WASHINGTON AVE ROYAL OAK MI 48067 (810) 414-7177

ARRAND MODELING SCHOOL 13344 WENWOOD DR SAGINAW MI 48603 (517) 790-9930

A-1 ASSOCIATED MODELS INC 17250 W 12 MILE RD SOUTHFIELD MI 48076 (810) 559-9150

AAA AGENCY-POWERS MODEL 16250 NORTHLAND DR # 239 SOUTHFIELD MI 48075 (810) 569-2247

AVENUE MODELS INC   29425 NORTHWESTERN HWY SOUTHFIELD MI 48034 (810) 358-2302

ETERNAL MANAGEMENT 2909 NORTHWESTERN HWY SOUTHFIELD MI 48034 (810) 443-2170

JOHN ROBERT POWERS SCHOOL 16250 NORTHLAND DR # 239 SOUTHFIELD MI 48075 (810) 569-1234

UFO TALENT & PRODUCTIONS 2009 ORCHARD LAKE RD SYLVAN LAKE MI 48320 (810) 332-0800

AFFILIATED MODELS INC 1680 CROOKS RD # 200 TROY MI 48084 (810) 244-8770

BARBIZON SCHOOL 6230 ORCHARD LAKE RD # 110 WEST BLOOMFIELD MI 48322 (810) 855-0251

Minnesota

PRO IMAGE 9062 LYNDALE AVE S BLOOMINGTON MN 55420 (612) 884-4499

JOHN CASABLANCAS CTR 7701 YORK AVE S EDINA MN 55435 (612) 835-5512

MODEL CONNECTION 6950 FRANCE AVE S EDINA MN 55435 (612) 920-9456

ZOOM AGENCY 7701 YORK AVE S EDINA MN 55435 (612) 835-4277

HOFFMAN TALENT AGENCY EXCELSIOR MN 55331 (612) 470-9855

NUTS 1355 OREGON AVE N GOLDEN VALLEY MN 55427 (612) 544-9450

MODEL & TALENT MANAGEMENT 2785 WHITE BEAR AVE N MAPLEWOOD MN 55109 (612) 777-8031

ACME TALENT AGENCY 708 N 1ST ST MINNEAPOLIS MN 55401 (612) 338-6393

CARYN MODEL & TALENT AGENCY 100 N 6TH ST # 270B MINNEAPOLIS MN 55403 (612) 349-3600

CREATIVE CASTING INC 10 S 5TH ST MINNEAPOLIS MN 55402 (612) 375-0525

CREATURE TALENT AGENCY 3411 ST PAUL AVE MINNEAPOLIS MN 55416 (612) 925-6011

ELEANOR MOORE MODEL & TALENT 1610 W LAKE ST MINNEAPOLIS MN 55408 (612) 827-3823

KIMBERLY FRANSON MODEL/ACTOR 430 N 1ST AVE # 410 MINNEAPOLIS MN 55401 (612) 338-1605

MODEL'S RESOURCE CTR 25 UNIVERSITY AVE SE MINNEAPOLIS MN 55414 (612) 379-3191

NATIONAL TALENT ASSOC 12 S 6TH ST MINNEAPOLIS MN 55402 (612) 338-4500

PORTFOLIO 1 MODELS & TALENTS 33 S 5TH ST # 120 MINNEAPOLIS MN 55402 (612) 338-5800

SUSAN WEHMANN MODELS & TALENT 1128 HARMON PL # 205 MINNEAPOLIS MN 55403 (612) 333-6393

IMAGE 1 PRO MODELING & ACTING 601 9TH AVE N ST CLOUD MN 56303 (320) 251-0101

LA TERESE IMAGE & MODELING 211 5TH AVE S ST CLOUD MN 56301 (320) 654-6053

MAREY MODELS & TALENT AGENCY 102 E ST GERMAIN ST ST CLOUD MN 56304 (320) 259-1304

NEW FACES MODELS & TALENTS INC 6301 WAYZATA BLVD ST LOUIS PARK MN 55416 (612) 544-8668

MEREDITH MODEL MANAGEMENT 555 7TH ST W ST PAUL MN 55102 (612) 298-9555

VOICE PLUS 1564 5TH ST WHITE BEAR LAKE MN 55110 (612) 426-9400

MISSOURI

ALEXANDRA & ASSOC 15928 KETTINGTON RD CHESTERFIELD MO 63017 (314) 391-1333

STAR MANAGEMENT 620 WOODLANDER DR JEFFERSON CITY MO 65101 (573) 634-7829

KAY MODELING & PHOTOGRAPHY 1201 W 7TH ST JOPLIN MO 64801 (417) 781-4540

AMERICAN ARTISTS AGENCY 1808 BROADWAY ST KANSAS CITY MO 64108 (816) 474-9988

EXPOSURE MODEL & TALENT 215 W 18TH ST KANSAS CITY MO 64108 (816) 842-4494

JOHN CASABLANCAS MODEL MGMT 330 W 47TH ST # 220 KANSAS CITY MO 64112 (816) 561-9400

MODEL & TALENT MANAGEMENT 330 W 47TH ST KANSAS CITY MO 64112 (816) 561-9967

MTC MODELS TALENT CHARM 4043 BROADWAY ST KANSAS CITY MO 64111 (816) 531-3223

PATRICIA STEVENS FASHION AGCY 4638 J C NICHOLS PKY KANSAS CITY MO 64112 (816) 531-3800

STRONG MODEL MANAGEMENT 3200 GILLHAM RD KANSAS CITY MO 64109 (816) 931-5140

TALENT UNLIMITED 4049 PENNSYLVANIA AVE KANSAS CITY MO 64111 (816) 561-9040

VOICES INC 3725 BROADWAY ST KANSAS CITY MO 64111 (816) 753-8255

DEBALINA MODELING 111 N MAIN ST # 107 KIRKSVILLE MO 63501 (816) 627-1717

ACTION TALENT 3825 S CAMPBELL AVE SPRINGFIELD MO 65807 (417) 883-2366

AUSTIN STROUP TALENT CNCTN 1736 E SUNSHINE ST SPRINGFIELD MO 65804 (417) 865-8815

NORMA'S MODELING SCHOOL & AGCY 3638 S CAMPBELL AVE SPRINGFIELD MO 65807 (417) 882-2436

BARBIZON MODELING AGENCY 7525 FORSYTH BLVD ST LOUIS MO 63105 (314) 863-1142

DELCIA AGENCY 7201 DELMAR BLVD ST LOUIS MO 63130 (314) 726-3223

DONNA BELLA INC 1627 LOCUST ST ST LOUIS MO 63103 (314) 231-7476

IMAGES OF ST LOUIS 715 OLD FRONTENAC SQ ST LOUIS MO 63131 (314) 993-0605

KIDS OF AMERICA 2344 LOUISIANA AVE ST LOUIS MO 63104 (314) 865-4222

MODEL MANAGEMENT 11815 MANCHESTER RD ST LOUIS MO 63131 (314) 773-6162

POWERS PROMOTIONS BY IOS 713 OLD FRONTENAC SQ ST LOUIS MO 63131 (314) 993-9339

PRIMA MODELS 522 S HANLEY RD ST LOUIS MO 63105 (314) 721-1235

QUANTUM FX 337 N EUCLID AVE ST LOUIS MO 63108 (314) 361-1151

TALENTPLUS-AFTRA/SAG 55 MARYLAND PLZ ST LOUIS MO 63108 (314) 367-5588

TOP OF THE LINE MODELING 1602 LOCUST ST ST LOUIS MO 63103 (314) 241-7791

MISSISSIPPI

Y M STUDIO 455 2ND ST BELMONT MS 38827 (601) 454-7787

STUDIO VOGUE MODEL MANAGEMENT HIGHWAY 45 N COLUMBUS MS 39701 (601) 328-3789

GO FOR IT MODEL MANAGEMENT CO 402 W PASCAGOULA ST JACKSON MS 39203 (601) 353-0049

JA CAR MODELING STUDIO 404 W PASCAGOULA ST JACKSON MS 39203 (601) 948-5553

AMERICA'S MISS INC 517 N 13TH AVE LAUREL MS 39440 (601) 425-0308

ALABAMA TALENT MANAGEMENT PO BOX 1331 PHILADELPHIA MS 39350 (205) 364-8700

STUDIO VOGUE BARNES CROSSING MALL TUPELO MS 38801 (601) 841-0152

MONTANA

CREATIVE WORLD MODELING 27 N 27TH ST BILLINGS MT 59101 (406) 259-9540

MONTANA MYSTIQUE TALENT AGENCY PO BOX 3244 BOZEMAN MT 59772 (406) 586-6099

WINSLOW STUDIO & GALLERY 16 S TRACY AVE BOZEMAN MT 59715 (406) 587-8826

MAXIE'S MODEL & TALENT AGENCY 401 HC CLANCY MT 59634 (406) 933-8461

NORTH CAROLINA

ARTISIANS AGENCY 58 HOLLAND ST ASHEVILLE NC 28801 (704) 253-3771

TALENT TREK AGENCY 46 HAYWOOD ST ASHEVILLE NC 28801 (704) 251-0173

BARBIZON MODELING 8318 PINEVILLE MATTHEWS RD CHARLOTTE NC 28226 (704) 544-1550

CAROLINA TALENT 227 W TRD ST CHARLOTTE NC 28202 (704) 332-3218

CAROLINA TALENT INC 312 RENSSELAER AVE CHARLOTTE NC 28203 (910) 665-9077

DIRECTIONS USA 206 E TREMONT AVE CHARLOTTE NC 28203 (704) 377-3151

FRANKLIN GROUP 222 E MOREHEAD ST CHARLOTTE NC 28202 (704) 333-8123

JTA TALENT AGENCY INC 820 EA BLVD CHARLOTTE NC 28203 (704) 377-5987

MODEL SHOPPE' 5701 EXECUTIVE CTR CHARLOTTE NC 28212 (704) 532-6577

PROFESSIONAL MODEL'S GUILD 1819 CHARLOTTE DR CHARLOTTE NC 28203 (704) 377-9299

STONE AGENCY 1819 CHARLOTTE DR CHARLOTTE NC 28203 (704) 377-9299

WILLIAM PETTIT AGENCY 401 EA BLVD CHARLOTTE NC 28203 (704) 343-4922

CITIES CLASSIC MODEL 821 CLOVERLEAF PLZ CONCORD NC 28025 (704) 786-2256

KICK 277 MODELING AGENCY 210 W MAIN ST DALLAS NC 28034 (704) 922-5425

TRIANGLE TALENT & PRODUCTION 3020 PICKETT RD DURHAM NC 27705 (919) 489-4477

DISCOVERY SCHOOL 103 S MCPHERSON CHURCH RD FAYETTEVILLE NC 28303 (910) 867-3337

DIRECTIONS USA 3717 W MARKET ST GREENSBORO NC 27403 (910) 292-2800

MARILYN'S INC 601 NORWALK ST GREENSBORO NC 27407 (910) 292-5950

RICK'S TALENT & MODELING AGCY 806 SUMMIT AVE GREENSBORO NC 27405 (910) 379-0033

TALENT CONNECTION 338 N ELM ST GREENSBORO NC 27401 (910) 274-2499

NANSEE'S PROMOTIONAL AGENCY RR 3 HENDERSON NC 27536 (919) 492-1554

IMAGE & FASHION ACADEMY 580 12TH AVE NE HICKORY NC 28601 (704) 327-3349

MODELS UNLIMITED 329 13TH AVE NW HICKORY NC 28601 (704) 322-8553

NEW VOICE MUSIC & TALENT 212 E MAIN ST LINCOLNTON NC 28092 (704) 735-4141

KIRYA BICHETTE 163 STRADE ST MATTHEWS NC 28105 (704) 846-5744

BARBIZON SCHOOL OF MODELING 4109 WAKE FOREST RD # 400 RALEIGH NC 27609 (919) 876-8201

BIZO'N TALENT MANAGEMENT 4109 WAKE FOREST RD # 400 RALEIGH NC 27609 (919) 876-6475

ESTEEM AGENCY 3820 MERTON DR RALEIGH NC 27609 (919) 787-7766

ARTISTS RESOURCE AGENCY 174 HUNTERS GLEN DR SUMMERFIELD NC 27358 (910) 349-6167

NANCY WATSON AGENCY PO BOX 557 WAXHAW NC 28173 (704) 843-1219

BONTALENT 2018 PRINCESS PLACE DR WILMINGTON NC 28405 (910) 343-0445

CORNUCOPIA AGENCY INC 2740 VANCE ST WILMINGTON NC 28412 (910) 452-0084

DELIA MODEL MANAGEMENT 2422 WRIGHTSVILLE AVE WILMINGTON NC 28403 (910) 343-1753

FINCANNON & ASSOC 201 N FRONT ST WILMINGTON NC 28401 (910) 251-1500

JTA TALENT AGENCY INC 16 S FRONT ST WILMINGTON NC 28401 (910) 762-7262

MAULTSBY MODEL & TALENT AGENCY 1213 CULBRETH DR WILMINGTON NC 28405 (910) 256-3130

MJM TALENT REPRESENTATIVE 2011 CAROLINA BEACH RD WILMINGTON NC 28401 (910) 251-3734

SHOW PEOPLE TALENT 201 N FRONT ST WILMINGTON NC 28401 (910) 815-0131

WILLIAM PETTIT AGENCY 23 N FRONT ST WILMINGTON NC 28401 (910) 762-1933

JOHNSON WEST TALENT 245 N HAWTHORNE RD WINSTON SALEM NC 27104 (910) 722-9099

NORTH DAKOTA

ACADEMIE 220 1 4 BROADWAY FARGO ND 58102 (701) 235-8132

NEW ENGLAND

BREAK A PAW TALENT AGENCY 512 S 7TH ST # 200 LINCOLN NE 68508 (402) 477-8722

IMAGINE MODELING TALENT AGENCY 512 S 7TH ST # 200 LINCOLN NE 68508 (402) 475-4624

NOIR BLANC TALENT CORP 3701 O ST # 202G LINCOLN NE 68510 (402) 475-1855

REAL PEOPLE 824 P ST # 103 LINCOLN NE 68508 (402) 438-2833

ACTORS ETC LTD 9773 LAFAYETTE PLZ OMAHA NE 68114 (402) 391-3153

INTERNATIONAL SCHOOL-MODELING 8602 CASS ST OMAHA NE 68114 (402) 399-8787

NANCY BOUNDS SCHOOL-AGENCY 11915 PIERCE PLZ OMAHA NE 68144 (402) 558-9292

NEW HAMPSHIRE

ROYAL MODELING ACADEMIE 48 E DERRY RD EAST DERRY NH 03041 (603) 432-8257

CINDERELLA MODELING STUDIO 9 BROOK ST MANCHESTER NH 03104 (603) 627-4125

NEW ENGLAND MODELS GROUP 175 CANAL ST MANCHESTER NH 03101 (603) 624-0555

VOGUE MODELING AGENCY 200 BEDFORD ST MANCHESTER NH 03101 (603) 622-5661

WEBB MODEL MANAGEMENT 1 MIDDLE ST PORTSMOUTH NH 03801 (603) 430-9334

PROFILE MODEL AGENCY 50 NORTHWESTERN DR SALEM NH 03079 (603) 893-2414

NEW JERSEY

ACTING WORKSHOP-WEIST-BARRON 2921 ATLANTIC AVE ATLANTIC CITY NJ 08401 (609) 347-0074

CLASSIC MODEL & TALENT MGMT 87 S FINLEY AVE BASKING RIDGE NJ 07920 (908) 766-6663

*TLW MODELING & PROMOTIONS 188 BALDWIN BLOOMFIELD NJ 07003 (201) 680-9859

NEW TALENT MANAGEMENT 590 RT 70 BRICK NJ 08723 (908) 477-3355

MODELS ON THE MOVE 1200 E MARLTON PIKE # 6 CHERRY HILL NJ 08034 (609) 667-1060

TALENT MARKETING INC 1135 CLIFTON AVE CLIFTON NJ 07013 (201) 779-0700

EMPIRE CASTING 3 MERRY LN EAST HANOVER NJ 07936 (201) 428-6009

CONSTANZA MODELING CTR 339 MORRIS AVE ELIZABETH NJ 07208 (908) 353-1188

LIGHTS CAMERA ACTION 15 GLORIA LN FAIRFIELD NJ 07004 (201) 227-3991

NATIONAL TALENT ASSOC INC 186 FAIRFIELD RD FAIRFIELD NJ 07004 (201) 575-7300

STAR TRAK REHERSAL STUDIOS 15 GLORIA LN FAIRFIELD NJ 07004 (201) 575-5877

UNIQUE MODELING AGENCY 30 TWO BRIDGES RD FAIRFIELD NJ 07004 (201) 227-0003

HOLLYWOOD IMAGE AGENCY 2011 LEMOINE AVE FORT LEE NJ 07024 (201) 944-1228

L & M MODELING INC 232 BLVD HASBROUCK HTS NJ 07604 (201) 288-2253

BARBIZON SCHOOL OF MODELING 300 RARITAN AVE HIGHLAND PARK NJ 08904 (908) 846-3800

SCREEN TEST USA 1700 GALLOPING HILL RD KENILWORTH NJ 07033 (908) 298-8000

MC CULLOUGH MODELS INC 8 S HANOVER AVE MARGATE CITY NJ 08402 (609) 822-2222

JO ANDERSON MODELING SCHOOL 882 N RT 73 MARLTON NJ 08053 (609) 596-7200

SUSAN ANDERSON MODELING AGENCY 1 GREENTREE CTR MARLTON NJ 08053 (609) 988-5460

NATIONAL TALENT ASSOC 2 S CTR ST MERCHANTVILLE NJ 08109 (609) 663-8500

CLERI MODEL MANAGEMENT CORP 402 MAIN ST METUCHEN NJ 08840 (908) 632-9544

AXIS MODELS & TALEN INC 20 CHURCH ST MONTCLAIR NJ 07042 (201) 783-4900

CAMELOT MODELING CONSULTANTS 20 CHURCH ST MONTCLAIR NJ 07042 (201) 509-8522

BENNIE ISSAMADEEN INC 51 CLIFTON AVE NEWARK NJ 07104 (201) 483-1727

MEADOWLANDS MODELING INC 7601 BROADWAY NORTH BERGEN NJ 07047 (201) 869-3107

PRISCILLA PARKER TALENT ACTION 2317 BAY AVE OCEAN CITY NJ 08226 (609) 399-7065

MODEL TEAM 55 CENTRAL AVE OCEAN GROVE NJ 07756 (908) 988-3648

BARBIZON SCHOOL OF MODELING 80 BROAD ST RED BANK NJ 07701 (908) 842-6161

PARK WEST MODEL & TALENT AGCY 20 W RIDGEWOOD AVE RIDGEWOOD NJ 07450 (201) 447-3335

COVER GIRL STUDIO 630 KINDERKAMACK RD RIVER EDGE NJ 07661 (201) 261-2042

MEREDITH MODEL MANAGEMENT 10 FURLER ST TOTOWA NJ 07512 (201) 812-0122

BARBIZON SCHOOL OF MODELING 2103 WHITEHORSE MERC RD TRENTON NJ 08619 (609) 586-3310

CALIFORNIA MODELING SCHOOL 937 BRUNSWICK AVE TRENTON NJ 08638 (609) 393-3323

DELL MODELING & MANAGEMENT CTR 312 GANTTOWN RD TURNERSVILLE NJ 08012 (609) 589-4099

CHRISTINE MODELS & CASTING 19 CASTLES DR WAYNE NJ 07470 (201) 904-0300

MORTON RAYFIELD UNLIMITED INC 659 EAGLE ROCK AVE WEST ORANGE NJ 07052 (201) 736-6966

SANDI STEWART MODEL-TALENT 659 EAGLE ROCK AVE WEST ORANGE NJ 07052 (201) 736-6984

MISS AMERICAN PETITE INC 59 MILL POND RD WEST PATERSON NJ 07424 (201) 890-9191

PATRICIA RAINEY INC 175 FOX HOLLOW RD WYCKOFF NJ 07481 (201) 652-1990

PRESTIGE MODELS INC 291 FRANKLIN AVE WYCKOFF NJ 07481 (201) 891-8600

New Mexico

APPLAUSE TALENT AGENCY 225 SAN PEDRO DR NE ALBUQUERQUE NM 87108 (505) 262-9733

ASPIRE MODELING AGENCY & MGMT 238 HORTON LN NW ALBUQUERQUE NM 87114 (505) 898-6980

CASTING CENTER 1209 MOUNTAIN RD PL NE ALBUQUERQUE NM 87110 (505) 262-2360

CIMARRON TALENT AGENCY 10605 CASADOR DEL OSO NE ALBUQUERQUE NM 87111 (505) 292-2314

DOUBLE TAKE MODEL & TAL 6921 MONTGOMERY BLVD NE ALBUQUERQUE NM 87109 (505) 880-1095

EATON AGENCY INC 3636 HIGH ST NE ALBUQUERQUE NM 87107 (505) 344-3149

I REHEARSAL STUDIOS 9928 BELL AVE SE ALBUQUERQUE NM 87123 (505) 294-2211

JOHN ROBERT POWERS 2021 SAN MATEO BLVD NE ALBUQUERQUE NM 87110 (505) 266-5677

MANNEQUIN AGENCY 2021 SAN MATEO BLVD NE ALBUQUERQUE NM 87110 (505) 266-6823

PHOENIX AGENCY 6400 UPTOWN BLVD NE ALBUQUERQUE NM 87110 (505) 881-1209

SOUTH OF SANTA FE 6921 MONTGOMERY BLVD NE ALBUQUERQUE NM 87109 (505) 880-8550

SOUTHWEST MODELS 218 E APACHE ST FARMINGTON NM 87401 (505) 325-5449

AESTHETICS MODELING & TALENT 489 CAMINO DON MIGUEL # A SANTA FE NM 87501 (505) 982-5884

CHARACTERS RR 9 BOX 73HH SANTA FE NM 87505 (505) 982-9729

NEVADA

A BASKOW TALENT AGENCY & ASSOC 2948 E RUSSELL RD LAS VEGAS NV 89120 (702) 733-7818

ANNE O'BRIANT AGENCY 4528 W CHARLESTON BLVD LAS VEGAS NV 89102 (702) 870-4499

BASS CREATIVE BOOKINGS 6188 S SANDHILL RD LAS VEGAS NV 89120 (702) 898-2277

BLUE DIAMOND TALENT AGENCY 7225 BERMUDA RD LAS VEGAS NV 89119 (702) 263-5724

CHARM UNLIMITED INC 880 E SAHARA AVE # 106 LAS VEGAS NV 89104 (702) 735-2335

CLASSIC MODELS LTD 3305 SPRING MOUNTAIN RD LAS VEGAS NV 89102 (702) 367-1444

CONVENTION EASE 3720 W DESERT INN RD LAS VEGAS NV 89102 (702) 365-1057

CREATIVE CASTING & ACTING 900 KAREN AVE LAS VEGAS NV 89109 (702) 737-0611

CREATIVE CONCEPTS 3135 INDUSTRIAL RD # 212 LAS VEGAS NV 89109 (702) 792-4111

FARRINGTON PRODUCTIONS INC 4350 ARVILLE ST # 27 LAS VEGAS NV 89103 (702) 362-3000

GEARY RINDELS ENTERPRISES 1921 SCENIC SUNRISE DR LAS VEGAS NV 89117 (702) 233-3600

HOLIDAY MODELS INC 900 E DESERT INN RD # 101 LAS VEGAS NV 89109 (702) 735-7353

JOHN CASABLANCAS MODEL & TLNT 2080 E FLAMINGO RD LAS VEGAS NV 89119 (702) 733-8140

JUDY VENN & ASSOC 3401 W CHARLESTON BLVD LAS VEGAS NV 89102 (702) 259-4494

LAS VEGAS MODELS 2255 RENAISSANCE DR LAS VEGAS NV 89119 (702) 737-1800

LENZ AGENCY PEOPLE WITH TALENT 1591 E DESERT INN RD LAS VEGAS NV 89109 (702) 733-6888

M MODELS 1555 E FLAMINGO RD # 436 LAS VEGAS NV 89119 (702) 737-8411

MATCH MODELS 1555 E FLAMINGO RD LAS VEGAS NV 89119 (702) 792-8320

MODELZAAR AGENCY 3135 INDUSTRIAL RD LAS VEGAS NV 89109 (702) 792-4118

NEW IMAGE MODELS 1600 E DESERT INN RD LAS VEGAS NV 89109 (702) 731-4872

NOUVELLE TALENT MANAGEMENT 4053 SPRING MOUNTAIN RD LAS VEGAS NV 89102 (702) 252-0024

PARKS PEOPLE 50 S JONES BLVD LAS VEGAS NV 89107 (702) 870-0555

PREMIERE MODELS 2700 STATE ST # 18 LAS VEGAS NV 89109 (702) 369-2003

SPECTRUM CASTING 8068 W SAHARA AVE LAS VEGAS NV 89117 (702) 433-9011

STARS UNLIMITED 2450 CHANDLER AVE LAS VEGAS NV 89120 (702) 795-8040

STARWEST INTERNATIONAL INC 125 E RENO AVE # 17 LAS VEGAS NV 89119 (702) 795-7091

TALENT QUEST INTERACTIVE 6260 STEVENSON WAY LAS VEGAS NV 89120 (702) 456-6335

THORNDIKE & ASSOC 3238 E OQUENDO RD LAS VEGAS NV 89120 (702) 454-9334

VOGUE MODELING AGENCY 3753 HOWARD HUGHES PKY # 121 LAS VEGAS NV 89109 (702) 792-1333

DEAN SCOTT MANAGEMENT 612 HUMBOLDT ST RENO NV 89509 (702) 322-3544

J F MANAGEMENT INC 280 ISLAND AVE RENO NV 89501 (702) 786-9997

NEVADA CASTING GROUP INC 100 WASHINGTON ST RENO NV 89503 (702) 322-8187

NEW YORK

BARBARA THOMAS MODELING SCHOOL 11 COMPUTER DR W ALBANY NY 12205 (518) 458-7849

BARBIZON MODELING 1991 CENTRAL AVE ALBANY NY 12205 (518) 456-6713

NEW ENGLAND MODELS 252 LARK ST ALBANY NY 12210 (518) 433-1281

PARAGON MODELING & TALENT 225 DEER PARK AVE BABYLON NY 11702 (516) 422-8900

FRESH FACES MANAGEMENT 2911 CARNATION AVE BALDWIN NY 11510 (516) 223-0034

STAR TIME MANAGEMENT 31 INDIANA AVE BAY SHORE NY 11706 (516) 665-5400

ELAINE GORDON MODEL 2557 LEFFERTS PL BELLMORE NY 11710 (516) 679-5850

THEATRE INTERNATIONAL INC 1517 E 172ND ST BRONX NY 10472 (718) 842-8570

UJAMAA BLACK THEATRE CO 1133 OGDEN AVE BRONX NY 10452 (718) 992-0938

BARBIZON SCHOOL OF MODELING 415 7TH AVE BROOKLYN NY 11215 (718) 230-0550

MODELS ASSOCIATION BOOKING SVC 241 WAVERLY AVE BROOKLYN NY 11205 (718) 857-6731

CONWELL CAREER CENTRE 2 SYMPHONY CIR BUFFALO NY 14201 (716) 884-0763

JENERO INC 1807 ELMWOOD AVE BUFFALO NY 14207 (716) 876-1280

JUNE 2 MODEL & TALENT AGENCY 143 ALLEN ST BUFFALO NY 14201 (716) 883-0700

TAC MODEL & TALENT MANAGEMENT 3095 ELMWOOD AVE BUFFALO NY 14217 (716) 874-5155

WRIGHT MODELING AGENCY 3719 UNION RD # 217 CHEEKTOWAGA NY 14225 (716) 685-5746

NORTH SHORE STUDIOS INC 216 ELWOOD RD EAST NORTHPORT NY 11731 (516) 261-5527

SCREEN TEST INC 101 EXECUTIVE BLVD ELMSFORD NY 10523 (914) 347-6500

BLACKWOOD-STEELE INC 694 MACEDON CTR FAIRPORT NY 14450 (716) 425-7099

NEXUS PERSONAL MANAGEMENT INC 694 MACEDON CTR FAIRPORT NY 14450 (716) 425-1306

A UNIQUE MODEL SVC 1919 RT 110 FARMINGDALE NY 11735 (516) 293-7017

MODEL MERCHANDISING INTL INC 164 MILBAR BLVD FARMINGDALE NY 11735 (516) 694-0005

TALENT ON LOCATION 2206 RT 9 FISHKILL NY 12524 (914) 897-2669

CAMERA TWO MODELING & ACTING 7206 AUSTIN ST FLUSHING NY 11375 (718) 793-3661

NEXT STOP IDEALS 6115 MYRTLE AVE FLUSHING NY 11385 (718) 497-7628

CHRISTINA MODELS 55 S BERGEN PL # 4E FREEPORT NY 11520 (516) 868-5932

MORGAN MANAGEMENT 315 W SUNRISE HWY # 2 FREEPORT NY 11520 (516) 546-3554

MARGO GEORGE MODELING 159 W MAIN ST GOSHEN NY 10924 (914) 294-8144

MIRROR MODEL & TALENT AGENCY 607 MIDDLE NECK RD GREAT NECK NY 11023 (516) 826-4788

JOYCE AGENCY INC 370 HARRISON AVE HARRISON NY 10528 (914) 835-1123

MCA THE MODEL & TALENT AGCY 11 CAMELIA PL HAUPPAUGE NY 11788 (516) 864-6320

STAR MAKERS INC 31 CARPENTER LN HAUPPAUGE NY 11788 (516) 348-7521

OMNIPOP INC TALENT AGENCIES 55 W OLD COUNTRY RD HICKSVILLE NY 11801 (516) 937-6011

JENNIFER MODELS INC AGENCY 168 MAIN ST HUNTINGTON NY 11743 (516) 385-4924

B F MODELING & ADVERTISING STD 825 E JERICHO TPKE HUNTINGTON STA NY 11746 (516) 673-0200

PRETTY PEOPLE MODEL MANAGEMENT 366 N BROADWAY JERICHO NY 11753 (516) 939-2899

HOLLYWOOD IMAGE PHOTO STUDIO 247 W MONTAUK HWY LINDENHURST NY 11757 (516) 226-0356

TIFFANY'S SHOOTING STARS 145 E SUNRISE HWY LINDENHURST NY 11757 (516) 888-1583

BARBIZON MODELING 117 METROPOLITAN PARK DR LIVERPOOL NY 13088 (315) 457-7580

INTERNATIONAL SHOW BUSINESS 3185 30TH ST LONG ISLAND CITY NY 11106 (718) 956-1268

ERNIE MARTINELLI MANAGEMENT 491 UNION VALLEY RD MAHOPAC NY 10541 (914) 628-9005

VOGUE MODELS MANAGEMENT 22 BEAUMONT DR MELVILLE NY 11747 (516) 643-9008

MARY THERESE FRIEL INC 1251 PITTSFORD MENDON RD MENDON NY 14506 (716) 624-5510

ELAINE GORDON MODEL MANAGEMENT 2942 HARBOR RD MERRICK NY 11566 (516) 623-7736

A L MODELS TALENT MANAGEMENT 168 5TH AVE NEW YORK NY 10010 (212) 366-6390

A P VARIETY TALENT AGENCY 175 5TH AVE NEW YORK NY 10010 (212) 582-1734

A PLUS MODELS LTD 311 W 43RD ST # 906 NEW YORK NY 10036 (212) 633-1990

ABBY HOFFER ENTERPRISES 223 E 48TH ST # A NEW YORK NY 10017 (212) 935-6350

ABRAMS ARTIST & ASSOC LTD 420 MADISON AVE NEW YORK NY 10017 (212) 935-8980

ACTION MODELS INC 134 W 32ND ST NEW YORK NY 10001 (212) 279-3720

ACTORS GROUP AGENCY 157 W 57TH ST # 604 NEW YORK NY 10019 (212) 245-2930

AGENTS FOR THE ARTS INC 203 W 23RD ST # 3 NEW YORK NY 10011 (212) 229-2562

AL ROTH THEATRICAL PRODUCTIONS 333 CENTRAL PARK W NEW YORK NY 10025 (212) 865-0241

ALAN WILLIG & ASSOC INC 47 HORATIO ST NEW YORK NY 10014 (212) 645-9400

ALLAN ALBERT PRODUCTIONS INC 561 BROADWAY # 10C NEW YORK NY 10012 (212) 966-8881

ALLIANCE TALENT INC 1501 BROADWAY NEW YORK NY 10036 (212) 840-6868

AMBROSIO MORTIMER & ASSOC INC 165 W 46TH ST # 1214 NEW YORK NY 10036 (212) 719-1677

AMERICAN MODEL MANAGEMENT CORP 155 SPRING ST NEW YORK NY 10012 (212) 941-5858

AMERICAN-INTERNATIONAL TALENT 303 W 42ND ST NEW YORK NY 10036 (212) 245-8888

ANDREADIS TALENT AGENCY 119 W 57TH ST # 711 NEW YORK NY 10019 (212) 315-0303

ANN WRIGHT REPRESENTATIVES 165 W 46TH ST # 1105 NEW YORK NY 10036 (212) 764-6770

BANTA CATALOG & COMMERCIAL GRP 6 E 43RD ST NEW YORK NY 10017 (212) 922-1066

BARBIZON MODELING AGENCY 15 PENN PLZ NEW YORK NY 10001 (212) 239-1110

BARRY HAFT BROWN ARTISTS AGENCY 165 W. 46TH ST NEW YORK NY 10036 (212) 869-9310

BAUMAN HILLER & ASSOC AGENCY 250 W 57TH ST # 2223 NEW YORK NY 10107 (212) 757-0098

BEAUTIFUL PEOPLE UNLIMITED 1841 BROADWAY # 1000 NEW YORK NY 10023 (212) 765-7793

BETHANN MANAGEMENT CO 36 N MOORE ST NEW YORK NY 10013 (212) 925-2153

BETTER BODIES INC 22 W 19TH ST NEW YORK NY 10011 (212) 929-6789

BEVERLY ANDERSON AGENCIES 1501 BROADWAY NEW YORK NY 10036 (212) 944-7773

BIENSTOCK SPORTS 1740 BROADWAY # 24 NEW YORK NY 10019 (212) 307-1250

BONAFIDE MODEL MANAGEMENT 1123 BROADWAY NEW YORK NY 10010 (212) 691-6394

BOOKERS 150 5TH AVE NEW YORK NY 10011 (212) 645-9706

BOOKING GROUP 145 W 45TH ST # 8 NEW YORK NY 10036 (212) 869-9280

*BOSS MODELS INC 1 GANSEVOORT ST NEW YORK NY 10014 (212) 242-2444

BRET ADAMS LTD 448 W 44TH ST NEW YORK NY 10036 (212) 765-5630

BRYCO INC 222 E 44TH ST NEW YORK NY 10017 (212) 661-2782

CAROLINA MODELING WORKSHOP 414 W 53RD ST NEW YORK NY 10019 (212) 262-1292

*CARSON ADLER AGENCY 250 W 57TH ST # 808 NEW YORK NY 10107 (212) 307-1882

CARSON ORGANIZATION LTD 240 W 44TH ST NEW YORK NY 10036 (212) 221-1517

CE SOIR OF NEW YORK INC 120 E 32ND ST NEW YORK NY 10016 (212) 213-0505

CENTRAL CASTING 200 W 54TH ST NEW YORK NY 10019 (212) 582-4933

CHRISTIE OPPENHEIM ASSOC LTD 13 E 37TH ST # 5 NEW YORK NY 10016 (212) 213-4330

CITY MODEL MANAGEMENT PO BOX 526 NEW YORK NY 10021 (212) 628-1380

CLASSIQUE MODEL AGENCY 29 E 10TH ST NEW YORK NY 10003 (212) 533-8219

*CLICK MODEL MANAGEMENT 881 7TH AVE # 1013 NEW YORK NY 10019 (212) 315-2200

CLICK SHOWS 881 7TH AVE NEW YORK NY 10019 (212) 757-0420

CLUE MODEL MANAGEMENT INC 145 W 24TH ST NEW YORK NY 10011 (212) 843-4042

COLEMAN-ROSENBERG 155 E 55TH ST NEW YORK NY 10022 (212) 838-0734

COMPANY MODEL MANAGEMENT INC 270 LAFAYETTE ST # 1400 NEW YORK NY 10012 (212) 226-9190

CONRAD SHADLEN CORP 141 E 44TH ST # 804 NEW YORK NY 10017 (212) 370-9757

CONTEMPORARY CASTING LTD 260 W 52ND ST # 3F NEW YORK NY 10019 (212) 333-5958

CRYSTAL AGENCY 15 W 26TH ST NEW YORK NY 10010 (212) 686-2881

*CUNNINGHAM ESCOTT DIPENE 257 S PARK AVE # 9 NEW YORK NY 10010 (212) 477-1666

CUZZINS MANAGEMENT 250 W 57TH ST NEW YORK NY 10107 (212) 765-6559

CYD LEVIN & ASSOC 1501 BROADWAY # 406 NEW YORK NY 10036 (212) 840-9414

DBS NEW YORK 1 GANSEVOORT ST NEW YORK NY 10014 (212) 242-9111

DENNIS DONNA THEATRICAL AGENCY 170 W END AVE # 3K NEW YORK NY 10023 (212) 265-6920

DESIRE 232 MADISON AVE NEW YORK NY 10016 (212) 686-8777

DIRECTORS CO 311 W 43RD ST # 206 NEW YORK NY 10036 (212) 246-5877

DNA MODEL MANAGEMENT 145 HUDSON ST NEW YORK NY 10013 (212) 226-0080

DON BUCHWALD & ASSOC INC 10 E 44TH ST NEW YORK NY 10017 (212) 867-1070

DOUGLAS FAIRBANKS THEATRE 432 W 42ND ST NEW YORK NY 10036 (212) 239-4321

DUVA-FLACK ASSOC INC 200 W 57TH ST NEW YORK NY 10019 (212) 957-9600

EASTWOOD TALENT GROUP LTD 178 E 2ND ST NEW YORK NY 10009 (212) 645-2500

EDEN TALENT MANAGEMENT 280 MADISON AVE NEW YORK NY 10016 (212) 689-9555

*ELITE MODEL MANAGEMENT CORP 111 E 22ND ST NEW YORK NY 10010 (212) 529-9700

*ELITE RUNWAY INC 149 MADISON AVE # 201 NEW YORK NY 10016 (212) 686-5600

ELIZABETH ASSOCIATES INC 129 E 39TH ST NEW YORK NY 10016 (212) 683-7630

ENACT 135 W 29TH ST NEW YORK NY 10001 (212) 868-2173

ENACT 622 BROADWAY # 5A NEW YORK NY 10012 (212) 260-6150

ENTOURAGE TALENT ASSOC LTD 25 W 39TH ST NEW YORK NY 10018 (212) 997-1900

EPSTEIN WYCKOFF & ASSOC 311 W 43RD ST # 304 NEW YORK NY 10036 (212) 586-9110

*FIFI OSCARD AGENCY 24 W 40TH ST NEW YORK NY 10018 (212) 764-1100

FILM CINEMA CONSULTING 333 W 52ND ST NEW YORK NY 10019 (212) 307-7533

FLAUNT MODEL MANAGEMENT INC 114 E 32ND ST # 501 NEW YORK NY 10016 (212) 679-9011

FLICK EAST & WEST TALENTS INC 881 7TH AVE # 1110 NEW YORK NY 10019 (212) 307-1850

*FORD CHILDREN 344 E 59TH ST NEW YORK NY 10022 (212) 688-7613

*FORD MODEL INC 344 E 59TH ST NEW YORK NY 10022 (212) 688-8628

FOSTER-FELL/JFF MANAGEMENT INC 156 5TH AVE # 408 NEW YORK NY 10010 (212) 645-0300

FUNNY FACE TODAY INC 151 E 31ST ST # 24J NEW YORK NY 10016 (212) 686-4343

GAGE GROUP INC 315 W 57TH ST # 4H NEW YORK NY 10019 (212) 541-5250

GEM TALENT 630 9TH AVE NEW YORK NY 10036 (212) 489-2013

GENERATION MODEL MANAGEMENT 20 W 20TH ST NEW YORK NY 10011 (212) 727-7219

GERSH AGENCY NY INC 130 W 42ND ST # 2400 NEW YORK NY 10036 (212) 997-1818

GILCHRIST TALENT GROUP INC 630 W 39TH ST NEW YORK NY 10018 (212) 692-9166

*GILLA ROOS LTD 16 W 22ND ST # 3 NEW YORK NY 10010 (212) 727-7820

GIRL OH BOY 130 W 56TH ST NEW YORK NY 10019 (212) 957-2862

GOLDSTAR TALENT MANAGEMENT INC 850 7TH AVE NEW YORK NY 10019 (212) 315-4429

GONZALEZ MODEL & TALENT 112 E 23RD ST PH NEW YORK NY 10010 (212) 982-5626

*GRACE DE MARCO 350 5TH AVE, STE 3110 NEW YORK NY 10118 (212) 629-6404

GRAHAM AGENCY 311 W 43RD ST NEW YORK NY 10036 (212) 489-7730

GRAMERCY ONE ASSOC 111 E 22ND ST NEW YORK NY 10010 (212) 995-2575

GREENWICH FINANCIAL 67 WALL ST NEW YORK NY 10005 (212) 480-8217

GUY COLTER TALENT 224 W 54TH ST NEW YORK NY 10019 (212) 397-7736

*H V MODELS LTD 30 E 20TH ST NEW YORK NY 10003 (212) 228-0300

HANNS WOLTERS THEATRICAL AGCY 10 W 37TH ST # 3 NEW YORK NY 10018 (212) 714-0100

HARRY PACKWOOD TALENT LTD 250 W 57TH ST # 2012 NEW YORK NY 10107 (212) 586-8900

HEADLINE TALENT INC 1650 BROADWAY # 508 NEW YORK NY 10019 (212) 581-6900

HENDERSON HOGAN AGENCY INC 850 7TH AVE # 1003 NEW YORK NY 10019 (212) 765-5190

HUGHES MOSS CASTING LTD 311 W 43RD ST # 700 NEW YORK NY 10036 (212) 307-6690

HWA TALENT REPRESENTATIVE 36 E 22ND ST NEW YORK NY 10010 (212) 529-4555

I'M NY MODEL MANAGEMENT INC 400 W BROADWAY NEW YORK NY 10012 (212) 941-1333

IMAGE & ESTEEM TEAM INC 325 W 45TH ST NEW YORK NY 10036 (212) 265-7845

*IMG MODELS 170 5TH AVE # 10 NEW YORK NY 10010 (212) 627-0400

INTERNATIONAL CREATIVE MGMT 40 W 57TH ST NEW YORK NY 10019 (212) 556-5600

INTERNATIONAL LATIN SHOWCASE 747 10TH AVE # 1 NEW YORK NY 10019 (212) 247-8199

INTERNATIONAL MODEL & TALENT 165 MADISON AVE # 4 NEW YORK NY 10016 (212) 696-5991

INTERNATIONAL TALENT GROUP 729 7TH AVE NEW YORK NY 10019 (212) 221-7878

*IRENE MARIE MODEL MANAGEMENT 400 W. BROADWAY NEW YORK NY 10012 (212) 941-1333

*IT TALENT 251 5TH AVE NEW YORK NY 10016 (212) 481-7220

*J MICHAEL BLOOM & ASSOC 233 PARK AVE S NEW YORK NY 10003 (212) 529-6500

J MITCHELL MANAGEMENT 440 PARK AVE S NEW YORK NY 10016 (212) 679-3550

*JAN J TALENT 365 W 34TH ST, 2ND FLOOR NEW YORK NY 10001 (212) 967-5265

JERRY KAHN INC 853 7TH AVE # 7C NEW YORK NY 10019 (212) 245-7317

JERRY KRAVAT ENTERTAINMENT SVC 404 PARK AVE S NEW YORK NY 10016 (212) 686-2200

JOEL PITT LTD 144 W 57TH ST NEW YORK NY 10019 (212) 765-6373

JOHN CASABLANCAS MOD & CAR CTR 111 E 22ND ST NEW YORK NY 10010 (516) 694-0005

*JORDAN GILL & DORNBAUM TALENT 156 5TH AVE # 711 NEW YORK NY 10010 (212) 463-8455

K L MANAGEMENT INC 1501 BROADWAY NEW YORK NY 10036 (212) 730-9500

KARIN MODEL/N.Y. 524 BROADWAY, STE 404 NEW YORK NY 10011 (212) 226-4100

KELLER LOUIS 235 W 44TH ST NEW YORK NY 10036 (212) 575-1633

KID'S POWER 161 W 16TH ST NEW YORK NY 10011 (212) 243-4269

LALLY TALENT AGENCY 630 9TH AVE NEW YORK NY 10036 (212) 974-8718

LANDY SOBA MANAGEMENT 211 W 53RD ST NEW YORK NY 10019 (212) 586-0123

LANTZ OFFICE 888 7TH AVE # 2500 NEW YORK NY 10106 (212) 586-0200

LATIN AMER THEATRE ENSEMBLE 172 E 104TH ST NEW YORK NY 10029 (212) 410-4582

LIFE STYLES 900 BROADWAY NEW YORK NY 10003 (212) 460-0920

LIONEL LARNER LTD 119 W 57TH ST NEW YORK NY 10019 (212) 246-3105

LISA BOOTH MANAGEMENT INC 145 W 45TH ST NEW YORK NY 10036 (212) 921-2114

LLOYD KOLMER ENTERPRISES 65 W 55TH ST NEW YORK NY 10019 (212) 582-4735

LOOKS INTERNATIONAL 40 HARRISON ST NEW YORK NY 10013 (212) 349-5133

LURE INTERNATIONAL TALENT GRP 915 BROADWAY NEW YORK NY 10010 (212) 260-9300

LYNN KRESSEL-CASTING 445 PARK AVE # 7 NEW YORK NY 10022 (212) 605-9122

LYONS GROUP 505 8TH AVE NEW YORK NY 10018 (212) 239-3539

MADISON TALENT GROUP 310 MADISON AVE NEW YORK NY 10017 (212) 922-9600

*MAX MEN 30 E 20TH ST NEW YORK NY 10003 (212) 228-0278

*MC DONALD RICHARDS INC 156 5TH AVE # 222 NEW YORK NY 10010 (212) 627-3100

MEG SIMON CASTING 1600 BROADWAY NEW YORK NY 10019 (212) 245-7670

MEGA MODEL MANAGEMENT 26 W 17TH ST NEW YORK NY 10011 (212) 366-4049

*METROPOLITAN MODEL MANAGEMENT 5 W UNION SQ # 5 NEW YORK NY 10003 (212) 989-0100

MIC-A-TAC MANAGEMENT & BOOKING 150 5TH AVE NEW YORK NY 10011 (212) 645-9787

MICHAEL HARTIG AGENCY LTD 156 5TH AVE NEW YORK NY 10010 (212) 929-1772

MICHAEL PEPINO CASTING 611 BROADWAY # 523 NEW YORK NY 10012 (212) 691-3600

MICHAEL THOMAS AGENCY INC 305 MADISON AVE NEW YORK NY 10017 (212) 867-0303

MISS CHIQUITITA INTL USA 314 W 53RD ST NEW YORK NY 10019 (212) 765-7907

MODEL & TALENT MANAGEMENT 415 7TH AVE NEW YORK NY 10001 (212) 239-6608

MODEL DEVELOPMENT INC 40 E 23RD ST NEW YORK NY 10010 (212) 353-0200

MODEL PROPERTIES 300 PARK AVE S NEW YORK NY 10010 (212) 889-9455

MODEL STYLE INC 119 W 23RD ST NEW YORK NY 10011 (212) 807-8642

MODELING ASSN OF AMERICA INTL 350 E 54TH ST NEW YORK NY 10022 (212) 753-1555

MODELS SERVICE AGENCY INC 570 7TH AVE # 702 NEW YORK NY 10018 (212) 944-8896

MOHMANER MODELING & ACTING 1309 LEXINGTON AVE NEW YORK NY 10128 (212) 996-3955

NEW YORK KIDS MODELS & TALENT 45 W 21ST ST NEW YORK NY 10010 (212) 807-0055

*NEXT MANAGEMENT CO 23 WATTS ST # 5 NEW YORK NY 10013 (212) 925-5100

NORMAN REICH AGENCY INC 1650 BROADWAY NEW YORK NY 10019 (212) 399-2881

NY LA TALENT FINDERS 49 W 9TH ST NEW YORK NY 10011 (212) 598-9150

*NYTRO INC 134 SPRING ST # 6A NEW YORK NY 10012 (212) 219-2300

ONE ON ONE PRODUCTIONS 126 W 23RD ST NEW YORK NY 10011 (212) 691-6000

OPHELIA DE VORE & ASSOC 350 5TH AVE NEW YORK NY 10118 (212) 629-6400

PACE THEATRICAL GROUP 1515 BROADWAY NEW YORK NY 10036 (212) 391-0555

PARADIGM 200 W 57TH ST NEW YORK NY 10019 (212) 246-1030

PARIS MODEL REPS INC 468 S PARK AVE # 1704 NEW YORK NY 10016 (212) 759-2841

*PARIS-USA MODELS 468 PARK AVE S NEW YORK NY 10016 (212) 683-9040

PARTS MODELS 500 E 77TH ST NEW YORK NY 10162 (212) 744-6123

PASARELA MODELING & TALENT LTD 231 W 29TH ST NEW YORK NY 10001 (212) 594-1043

*PAULINES MODEL MANAGEMENT 379 W BROADWAY NEW YORK NY 10012 (212) 941-6000

PEGGY HADLEY ENTERPRISES LTD 250 W 57TH ST # 2317 NEW YORK NY 10107 (212) 246-2166

PETER BEILINE AGENCY INC 230 PARK AVE # 923 NEW YORK NY 10169 (212) 949-9119

PETER STRAIN & ASSOC 1501 BROADWAY # 2900 NEW YORK NY 10036 (212) 391-0380

PGA INC 1650 BROADWAY # 711 NEW YORK NY 10019 (212) 586-1452

PHOENIX TALENT AGENCY INC 581 9TH AVE NEW YORK NY 10036 (212) 564-4206

PLUS WOMEN MODEL MGMT LTD 49 W 37TH ST NEW YORK NY 10018 (212) 997-1785

RACHAEL'S TOTZ N TEENZ MODEL 134 W 29TH ST NEW YORK NY 10001 (212) 967-3167

RICHARD CATALDI AGENCY 180 7TH AVE NEW YORK NY 10011 (212) 741-7450

ROGER PAUL AGENCY 581 9TH AVE # 3C NEW YORK NY 10036 (212) 268-0005

*ROGERS & LERMAN 645 5TH AVE # 5 NEW YORK NY 10022 (212) 935-2300

ROSENBERG & SEAMAN 51 E 42ND ST NEW YORK NY 10017 (212) 286-0009

ROTHMAN SHELLY 101 W 57TH ST # 11E NEW YORK NY 10019 (212) 246-2180

ROXY HOREN PERSONNEL MGMT 300 W 17TH ST NEW YORK NY 10011 (212) 206-1396

RUDGE-KAUFF ENTERPRISES 122 E 57TH ST # 2 NEW YORK NY 10022 (212) 755-5700

RYBIN TALENT MANGEMENT LTD 250 W 54TH ST NEW YORK NY 10019 (212) 247-4760

SAMES & ROLLNICK ASSOC LTD 250 W 57TH ST NEW YORK NY 10107 (212) 315-4434

SANDERS AGENCY 1204 BROADWAY # 306 NEW YORK NY 10001 (212) 779-3737

*SCHULLER TALENT NEW YORK KIDS 276 5TH AVE # 1001 NEW YORK NY 10001 (212) 532-6005

*SEMM 22 W 19TH ST NEW YORK NY 10011 (212) 627-5500

SHEPLIN ARTIST & ASSOC 160 5TH AVE NEW YORK NY 10010 (212) 647-1311

SHERWIN M GOLDMAN PRODUCTIONS 1501 BROADWAY NEW YORK NY 10036 (212) 575-9263

SHOWBIZ NEWS MODEL NEWS 40 E 34TH ST NEW YORK NY 10016 (212) 683-0244

SILK MODEL MANAGEMENT 252 W 29TH ST NEW YORK NY 10001 (212) 695-8550

SILVER MASSETTI & ASSOC AGENCY 145 W 45TH ST # 1204 NEW YORK NY 10036 (212) 391-4545

SKY MODEL MANAGEMENT INC 107 GREENE ST NEW YORK NY 10012 (212) 343-9339

SPECIAL ARTISTS AGENCY INC 111 E 22ND ST NEW YORK NY 10010 (212) 420-0200

STARS MODEL MANAGEMENT INC 303 E 60TH ST NEW YORK NY 10022 (212) 758-3545

STOCK MODEL MANAGEMENT 125 5TH AVE NEW YORK NY 10003 (212) 529-4372

*SWIFT KIDS/PLUS MODELS 49 W. 37TH ST PENTHOUSE NEW YORK NY 10018 (212)   997-1785

SYLVIA FAY CASTING 71 PARK AVE NEW YORK NY 10016 (212) 889-2626

TALENT CONSULTANTS INTL LTD 1560 BROADWAY # 1308 NEW YORK NY 10036 (212) 730-2701

TALENT MANAGEMENT 1501 BROADWAY NEW YORK NY 10036 (212) 730-1444

TALENT PARTNERS 115 W 18TH ST NEW YORK NY 10011 (212) 727-1800

TALENT REPRESENTATIVE INC 20 E 53RD ST # 2A NEW YORK NY 10022 (212) 752-1835

TERRIFIC TALENT ASSOC 419 S PARK AVE # 10 NEW YORK NY 10016 (212) 689-2800

TESTBOARD 34 E 39TH ST # 2A NEW YORK NY 10016 (212) 986-8100

THEATRE FOR A NEW AUDIENCE 154 CHRISTOPHER ST # 3D NEW YORK NY 10014 (212) 229-2819

THOMPSON MODEL AGENCY INC 50 W 34TH ST # 6C6 NEW YORK NY 10001 (212) 947-6711

TRANUM ROBERTSON 2 DAG HAMMARSKJOLD PLZ # 601 NEW YORK NY 10017 (212) 371-7500

TRIANGLE THEATRE CO 316 E 88TH ST NEW YORK NY 10128 (212) 860-7244

TRIBE MODEL MANAGEMENT 51 HUDSON ST NEW YORK NY 10013 (212) 406-1010

VAN DER VEER MODELS 400 E 57TH ST NEW YORK NY 10022 (212) 688-2880

VOICECASTING 1600 BROADWAY # 407 NEW YORK NY 10019 (212) 581-5575

W 2 MODELS 300 PARK AVE S NEW YORK NY 10010 (212) 473-1613

WATERS & NICOLOSI 1501 BROADWAY # 1305 NEW YORK NY 10036 (212) 302-8787

*WILHELMINA MODELS INC 300 S PARK AVE # 2 NEW YORK NY 10010 (212) 473-0700

*WILHELMINA RUNWAY DIV 300 S PARK AVE # 2 NEW YORK NY 10010 (212) 473-4312

*WILLIAM MORRIS AGENCY INC 1325 AVENUE THE AMERICAS NEW YORK NY 10019 (212) 586-5100

WILLIAM SCHILL AGENCY 250 W 57TH ST NEW YORK NY 10107 (212) 315-5919

WOMEN MODEL MANAGEMENT 107 GREENE ST NEW YORK NY 10012 (212) 334-7480

YOUNG TALENT INC 301 E 62ND ST NEW YORK NY 10021 (212) 308-0930

*ZOLI MANAGEMENT INC 3 W 18TH ST NEW YORK NY 10011 (212) 242-1500

410 MODELS 340 ROBINSON AVE NEWBURGH NY 12550 (914) 562-1478

HUDSON MODELING WORKSHOPS INC 74 N BROADWAY NYACK NY 10960 (914) 358-9400

AZETAH MODEL & TALENT MGMT INC 2851 CLOVER ST PITTSFORD NY 14534 (716) 387-0930

CHICKYS KIDS 2 WILSHIRE LN PLAINVIEW NY 11803 (516) 822-3333

U S MODEL-TALENT MANAGEMENT 250 GOODMAN ST N ROCHESTER NY 14607 (716) 244-0592

MODEL DEVELOPMENT 222 SUNRISE HWY ROCKVILLE CENTRE NY 11570 (516) 594-9200

FAME TALENT AGENCY 1242 ADRIENNE LN SEAFORD NY 11783 (516) 221-5981

ADELE'S KIDS 33 RUPERT AVE STATEN ISLAND NY 10314 (718) 494-5000

ALL TALENT MANAGEMENT 183 SHARPE AVE STATEN ISLAND NY 10302 (718) 447-4616

REAL PEOPLE MANAGEMENT 200 WEATHERVANE WAY SYRACUSE NY 13209 (315) 487-0618

JOANNE'S FASHION & CHARM 2204 PINNACLE DR UTICA NY 13501 (315) 797-6424

NATIONAL TALENT ASSOC INC 40 RAILROAD AVE VALLEY STREAM NY 11580 (516) 825-8707

ARIA'S NEW YORK MODELS 343 LITTLE JOHN WAY WEBSTER NY 14580 (716) 265-4328

BARBIZON MODEL AGENCY MONTAUK HWY & ROUTE 109 WEST BABYLON NY 11704 (516) 587-6100

BARBIZON SCHOOL OF MODELING 190 E POST RD WHITE PLAINS NY 10601 (914) 428-2030

TANNEN'S TALENT & MODELS LTD 77 TARRYTOWN RD WHITE PLAINS NY 10607 (914) 946-0900

FACES 6814 MAIN ST # 110 WILLIAMSVILLE NY 14221 (716) 634-5634

NEW FACES 6814 MAIN ST WILLIAMSVILLE NY 14221 (716) 632-7181

CLICK INTERNATIONAL AGENCY JONES QUARRY RD WOODSTOCK NY 12498 (914) 679-7357

WOODSTOCK YOUTH THEATRE INC 17 HEMLOCK LN WOODSTOCK NY 12498 (914) 679-1027

Ohio

AMERICA'S MOST BEAUTIFUL BABY 698 JOLSON AVE AKRON OH 44319 (330) 644-7660

BARBIZON SCHOOL OF MODELING 3296 W MARKET ST AKRON OH 44333 (330) 867-4110

PRO-MODEL MANAGEMENT 3296 W MARKET ST AKRON OH 44333 (330) 867-4125

PROTOCOL MODEL & TALENT 1969 N CLEVELAND MASSILLON RD AKRON OH 44333 (330) 666-6066

Z MODELS INC 1867 W MARKET ST # 1 AKRON OH 44313 (330) 869-5050

C B GROUP 564 W. TUSCARAWAS AVE, STE 401 BARBERTON OH 44203 (330) 848-8699

NORTH AMER SCHOLASTIC PAGEANT 218 31ST ST NW BARBERTON OH 44203 (330) 825-3315

OHIO'S ALL AMERICAN GIRL & BOY 218 31ST ST NW BARBERTON OH 44203 (330) 825-3315

MARSHA MODEL & TALENT AGENCY 118 W HIGH ST BRYAN OH 43506 (419) 636-5334

DIMENSIONS PLUS-SIZE MODEL 551 36TH ST., NW CANTON OH 44709 (330) 649-9809

WORLDWIDE MODEL & TALENT 1235 WHIPPLE AVE NW CANTON OH 44708 (330) 477-4227

BETTE MASSIE INC 8075 MCEWEN RD # 8071 CENTERVILLE OH 45458 (937) 435-3477

ASHLEY TALENT 128 E 6TH ST CINCINNATI OH 45202 (513) 554-4836

BARBIZON SCHOOL OF MODELING 8180 CORPORATE PARK DR CINCINNATI OH 45242 (513) 530-8100

CAM TALENT INC 1150 W 8TH ST CINCINNATI OH 45203 (513) 421-1795

CREATIVE TALENT 700 W PETE ROSE WAY CINCINNATI OH 45203 (513) 241-7827

GLORIA SUSTAR AGENCY 35 E 7TH ST CINCINNATI OH 45202 (513) 721-3737

HEYMAN HALPER TALENT AGENCY 3308 BROTHERTON RD CINCINNATI OH 45209 (513) 533-3113

JACK MORAN ALL STAR TALENT 5714 SCARBOROUGH DR CINCINNATI OH 45238 (513) 922-0621

JOHN CASABLANCAS MODELING 10680 MCSWAIN DR CINCINNATI OH 45241 (513) 733-8998

JUDY BARRICK MODELING & ACTING 7057 PADDISON RD CINCINNATI OH 45230 (513) 751-3030

KATHLEEN WELLMAN SCHOOL 128 E 6TH ST CINCINNATI OH 45202 (513) 345-2445

LILLIAN GALLOWAY MODELING ACNY 6047 MONTGOMERY RD CINCINNATI OH 45213 (513) 351-2700

O'CONNELL LAURA 2141 GILBERT AVE CINCINNATI OH 45206 (513) 281-8030

PROFESSIONAL MODELS ASSN 9475 KENWOOD RD CINCINNATI OH 45242 (513) 984-6508

SAVVY MODELS INTL AGENCY 270 NORTHLAND BLVD CINCINNATI OH 45246 (513) 771-2222

ABOUT FACE 8748 BRECKSVILLE RD # 223 CLEVELAND OH 44141 (216) 526-9493

BARBIZON CAREER CTR 6450 ROCKSIDE WOODS BLVD S CLEVELAND OH 44131 (216) 642-5445

D'AVILA MODEL & TALENT MGMT 4611 YORKSHIRE AVE CLEVELAND OH 44134 (216) 623-3443

DAVID & LEE TALENT CHECK-IN 1300 E 9TH ST CLEVELAND OH 44114 (216) 522-1300

J W HUNTER & ASSOC 2393 PROFESSOR AVE CLEVELAND OH 44113 (216) 522-1010

MELANGE MODELING 3130 MAYFIELD RD CLEVELAND OH 44118 (216) 371-9710

TAXI MODEL MANAGEMENT 1300 W 78TH ST CLEVELAND OH 44102 (216) 781-8294

ARLINGTON MODELS 5663 SHADOWBROOK DR COLUMBUS OH 43235 (614) 279-5881

CLINE & MOSIC TALENT AGENCY 1350 W 5TH AVE # 25 COLUMBUS OH 43212 (614) 488-1122

CREATIVE TALENT CO 1102 NEIL AVE COLUMBUS OH 43201 (614) 294-7827

DISCOVERY LIMITED 700 ACKERMAN RD # 600 COLUMBUS OH 43202 (614) 265-2243

G O INTL MODEL MANAGEMENT 1227 PENNSYLVANIA AVE COLUMBUS OH 43201 (614) 848-7887

GO INTERNATIONAL MODEL MGMT 6555 BUSCH BLVD COLUMBUS OH 43229 (614) 488-9091

GOENNER TALENT AGENCY 4700 REED RD COLUMBUS OH 43220 (614) 459-3582

JOHN ROBERT POWERS MODELING 5900 ROCHE DR COLUMBUS OH 43229 (614) 846-1046

L'ESPRIT MODELS MANAGEMENT INC 4807 EVANSWOOD DR COLUMBUS OH 43229 (614) 885-9752

MODEL & TALENT MANAGEMENT 6322 BUSCH BLVD COLUMBUS OH 43229 (614) 847-4043

NONI AGENCY FINISHING SCHOOL 172 E STATE ST COLUMBUS OH 43215 (614) 224-7217

VERWOO INTERNATIONAL 4790 E LIVINGSTON AVE COLUMBUS OH 43227 (614) 863-5764

PROFILES MODELING & TALENT 2152 FRONT ST CUYAHOGA FALLS OH 44221 (330) 945-4556

JO GOENNER TALENT AGENCY 10019 PARAGON RD DAYTON OH 45458 (937) 885-2595

SHARKEY AGENCY INC 1299 LYONS RD DAYTON OH 45458 (937) 434-4461

WILLA SINGER SCHOOL-MODELING 17 N MAIN ST DAYTON OH 45402 (937) 439-0220

AGENCY FOR PROFESSIONAL MODELS 612 JACQUELINE CT HOLLAND OH 43528 (419) 865-2232

KAY LA MANAGEMENT CORP 3030 COLUMBIA TRL LOVELAND OH 45140 (513) 336-7554

ALL STAR MANAGEMENT 1229 S PROSPECT ST MARION OH 43302 (614) 382-5939

RUNWAY AGENCY 21 W CHURCH ST NEWARK OH 43055 (614) 345-4444

A GOLDEN TOUCH TALENT AGENCY 8527 REFUGEE RD PICKERINGTON OH 43147 (614) 837-0629

EXPRESSION INTL MODEL MGMT 1720 JEFFERSON AVE TOLEDO OH 43624 (419) 241-9457

MARGARET O'BRIEN'S INTL 330 S REYNOLDS RD TOLEDO OH 43615 (419) 536-5522

TALMAR 316 N MICHIGAN ST TOLEDO OH 43624 (419) 241-5630

TRAQUE MODEL MANAGEMENT 2107 PARKWOOD AVE # 3 TOLEDO OH 43620 (419) 244-7363

RIGHT DIRECTION 6660 N HIGH ST WORTHINGTON OH 43085 (614) 848-3357

AMERITAL AGENCY LTD 1802 BELMONT AVE YOUNGSTOWN OH 44504 (330) 747-2566

LEMODELN MODEL & TALENT AGENCY 7536 MARKET ST YOUNGSTOWN OH 44512 (330) 758-4417

OKLAHOMA

SHOWTIME NATIONAL TALENT PO BOX 541 EDMOND OK 73083 (405) 359-8656

TEXOMA TALENT SEARCH SATELLITE HWY 70 N IDABEL OK 74745 (405) 286-2258

BOX TALENT 219 W BOYD ST NORMAN OK 73069 (405) 360-2263

ACCESS MODEL & TALENT AGENCY 6488 AVONDALE DR OKLAHOMA CITY OK 73116 (405) 943-8001

AMAZIN MODELING INC 6051 N BROOKLINE AVE OKLAHOMA CITY OK 73112 (405) 843-5583

DONNA LEIRD TALENT AGENCY 2856 NW 63RD ST OKLAHOMA CITY OK 73116 (405) 840-4340

HARRISON-GERS MODEL & TALENT 2624 W BRITTON RD OKLAHOMA CITY OK 73120 (405) 840-4515

JOHN CASABLANCAS MGMT 5009 N PENNSYLVANIA AVE OKLAHOMA CITY OK 73112 (405) 842-0000

MODEL & TALENT MGMT   5009 N PENNSYLVANIA AVE OKLAHOMA CITY OK 73112 405 8420090

OKLAHOMA TALENT & MODEL ASSN PO BOX 25593 OKLAHOMA CITY OK 73125 405 7322212

A'MAZIN MODELING SCHOOL 8137 E 63RD PL TULSA OK 74133 (918) 254-4190

JOHN CASABLANCAS MODELING CTR 5840 S MEMORIAL DR # 322 TULSA OK 74145 (918) 622-2525

LINDA LAYMAN AGENCY LTD 3546 E 51ST ST TULSA OK 74135 (918) 744-0888

MODEL & TALENT MANAGEMENT 5840 S MEMORIAL DR # 322 TULSA OK 74145 (918) 622-2593

SEAN RIDGWAY AGENCY 1350 E 15TH ST TULSA OK 74120 (918) 587-3131

TULSA TALENT AGENCY 2761 E SKELLY DR TULSA OK 74105 (918) 747-9246

OREGON

ABC KIDS-N-TEENS ARTS CTR 1144 WILLAGILLESPIE RD EUGENE OR 97401 (541) 485-6960

TALENT MANAGEMENT ASSOC 1574 COBURG RD # 143 EUGENE OR 97401 (541) 345-1525

HIGH PROFILES AGENCY 345 N BARTLETT ST # 202 MEDFORD OR 97501 (541) 770-8089

ABC KIDS-N-TEENS PERFORMING 3829 NE TILLAMOOK ST PORTLAND OR 97212 (503) 249-2945

ACADEMY ONE INC 700 SW TAYLOR ST # 222 PORTLAND OR 97205 (503) 227-4757

ACTORS ONLY 2510 SE BELMONT ST PORTLAND OR 97214 (503) 233-5073

CENTRAL EXTRAS CASTING 037 SW HAMILTON ST PORTLAND OR 97201 (503) 243-2468

CREATIVE ARTIST MANAGEMENT 909 SW ST CLAIR AVE PORTLAND OR 97205 (503) 241-2855

CUSICK'S TALENT AGENCY 1009 NW HOYT ST # 100 PORTLAND OR 97209 (503) 274-8555

EXTRAS ONLY 322 SW 5TH AVE # 231 PORTLAND OR 97204 (503) 227-6055

FANTASTIKA 1306 NW HOYT ST # 407 PORTLAND OR 97209 (503) 241-4912

JOHN CASABLANCAS MODELING 5440 SW WESTGATE DR # 350 PORTLAND OR 97221 (503) 297-7730

PRO MODELS INC 921 SW MORRISON ST # 301 PORTLAND OR 97205 (503) 228-5648

REEL KIDS INC 4004 SW KELLY AVE PORTLAND OR 97201 (503) 248-4565

ROSE CITY TALENT 239 NW 13TH AVE PORTLAND OR 97209 (503) 274-1005

SPORTS UNLIMITED INC 1991 NW UPSHUR ST PORTLAND OR 97209 (503) 227-3449

CINDERELLA'S SCHOOL-MODEL AGCY 317 NE CT ST UPPR LVL SALEM OR 97301 (503) 581-1073

DE FORE' IMAGE CONSULTING SCHL 147 LIBERTY ST NE SALEM OR 97301 (503) 316-9672

Pennsylvania

CHARTREUSE TALENT WORKSHOPS 801 N 12TH ST ALLENTOWN PA 18102 (610) 433-5448

IMAGE INTERNATIONAL 4959 HAMILTON BLVD ALLENTOWN PA 18106 (610) 391-9133

PRO MODEL MANAGEMENT 1107 UNION BLVD ALLENTOWN PA 18103 (610) 820-5359

STAR TALENT MANAGEMENT 1109 UNION BLVD # 2 ALLENTOWN PA 18103 (610) 770-1200

STAR PROMOTIONS 315 LOGAN BLVD ALTOONA PA 16602 (814) 942-9446

BARBIZON SCHOOL OF MODELING 18 GREENFIELD AVE ARDMORE PA 19003 (610) 649-9700

SCREEN TEST USA 130 PRESIDENTIAL BLVD BALA CYNWYD PA 19004 (610) 667-7600

SLICKIS MODEL & TALENT AGENCY 1777 WALTON RD BLUE BELL PA 19422 (215) 540-0440

ROSS TALENT INTL 502 WASHINGTON AVE BRIDGEVILLE PA 15017 (412) 221-2221

UPDIKE MODELING AGENCY 3920 MARKET ST CAMP HILL PA 17011 (717) 730-8718

DU BOIS COMMUNITY THEATER 335 S JARED ST DU BOIS PA 15801 (814) 375-8686

AJB MODEL & TALENT MGMT 2318 W 8TH ST ERIE PA 16505 (814) 456-6335

RIANA INC CAREER CTR 3930 W RIDGE RD ERIE PA 16506 (814) 835-3930

VISION MODEL & TALENT AGENCY 5120 W RIDGE RD ERIE PA 16506 (814) 833-7346

BORTNER THEATRICAL RR 3 BOX 248 GLEN ROCK PA 17327 (717) 235-2007

BARBIZON SCHOOL OF MODELING 1033 MACLAY ST HARRISBURG PA 17103 (717) 234-3277

FASHION MYSTIQUE MODELING IH 83 & UNION DEPOSIT RD HARRISBURG PA 17111 (717) 561-2099

MODELS N MOTION HUNTINGTON MILLS PA 18622 (717) 864-3876

RALYN TALENTS BORDNERSVILLE RD JONESTOWN PA 17038 (717) 865-3096

MAIN LINE MODELS 160 N GULPH RD KING OF PRUSSIA PA 19406 (610) 337-2689

PLAZA-7 MODELS & TALENT 160 N GULPH RD KING OF PRUSSIA PA 19406 (610) 337-2693

BOWMAN AGENCY 1040 WOODRIDGE BLVD LANCASTER PA 17601 (717) 898-7716

GREER LANGE ASSOC 7 GREAT VALLEY PKY MALVERN PA 19355 (610) 647-5515

MAIN LINE MODELS 1215 W BALTIMORE PIKE # 9 MEDIA PA 19063 (610) 565-5445

FOLIO FASHION MODELS 1 MONROEVILLE CTR MONROEVILLE PA 15146 (412) 372-8980

JOY ACADEMY OF MODELING 580 UNION SCHOOL RD MT JOY PA 17552 (717) 653-2133

CLICK MODELS OF PHILADELPHIA 157 WOODGATE LN PAOLI PA 19301 (610) 394-0900

PRESTIGE MODELING INC 10034 FRANKSTOWN RD PENN HILLS PA 15235 (412) 731-4810

ASKINS MODELS NEWMARKET SQUARE # 200 PHILADELPHIA PA 19147 (215) 925-7795

BOUNDARY PROMOTIONS 2333 FAIRMOUNT AVE PHILADELPHIA PA 19130 (215) 232-6102

CLARO MODELING 1513 W PASSYUNK AVE # 2 PHILADELPHIA PA 19145 (215) 465-7788

CREATIVE SOURCE MANAGEMENT INC 5510 GREENE ST PHILADELPHIA PA 19144 (215) 848-1445

CREATIVE SOURCE MANAGEMENT INC 5510 GREENE ST PHILADELPHIA PA 19144 (215) 848-1445

DOLORES DECK MANAGEMENT 3800 GREENACRES RD PHILADELPHIA PA 19154 (215) 637-1775

EXPRESSIONS MODELING & TALENT 110 CHURCH ST PHILADELPHIA PA 19106 (215) 923-4420

IRENE BAIRD ACTING STUDIO 2120 N 63RD ST PHILADELPHIA PA 19151 (215) 477-0425

JERRY SAMUELS AGENCY 5870 OXFORD AVE PHILADELPHIA PA 19149 (215) 537-9726

JOHN ROBERT POWERS AGENCY 1528 SPRUCE ST PHILADELPHIA PA 19102 (215) 732-4060

KARISMA INC 1229 CHESTNUT ST PHILADELPHIA PA 19107 (215) 988-0550

KATHY WICKLINE CASTING 1084 N DELWARE AVE PHILADELPHIA PA 19125 (215) 629-1180

MAY HEDGES CASTING 104 LOMBARD ST PHILADELPHIA PA 19147 (215) 829-9001

MICHAEL LEMON CASTING DIRECTRS 413 N 7TH ST PHILADELPHIA PA 19123 (215) 627-8927

MIDIRI INC 22 N 3RD ST PHILADELPHIA PA 19106 (215) 567-7770

NEW LEGENDS 608 W UPSAL ST PHILADELPHIA PA 19119 (215) 843-8036

PHILA CASTING CO 128 CHESTNUT ST PHILADELPHIA PA 19106 (215) 592-7575

PHILADELPHIA THEATRE CARAVAN 3700 CHESTNUT ST PHILADELPHIA PA 19104 (215) 898-6068

PLAYS & PLAYERS 1714 DELANCEY PL PHILADELPHIA PA 19103 (215) 735-0630

REINHARD MODEL & TALENT AGENCY 2021 ARCH ST PHILADELPHIA PA 19103 (215) 567-2008

STAPHEN DA POR MODELING AGENCY 1422 CHESTNUT ST PHILADELPHIA PA 19102 (215) 751-0315

ZODA MODELING AGENCY INC 1831 CHESTNUT ST PHILADELPHIA PA 19103 (215) 567-3607

A MODELS UNLIMITED 1701 BANKSVILLE RD PITTSBURGH PA 15216 (412) 343-7000

CYNTHIA'S 4801 MCKNIGHT RD PITTSBURGH PA 15237 (412) 367-3330

DOCHERTY CASTING 109 MARKET ST # 2 PITTSBURGH PA 15222 (412) 765-1400

DONNA BOLAJAC & CO 109 MARKET ST PITTSBURGH PA 15222 (412) 391-1005

JOHN CASABLANCAS MODELING CTR 777 PENN CTR # 750 PITTSBURGH PA 15235 (412) 829-7373

TALENT GROUP 2820 SMALLMAN ST PITTSBURGH PA 15222 (412) 471-8011

VAN ENTERPRISES 9600 PERRY HWY PITTSBURGH PA 15237 (412) 364-0411

JOHN CASABLANCAS MODEL 170 W GERMANTOWN PIKE PLYMOUTH MEETING PA 19462 (610) 278-7700

DONATELLI MODEL & CASTING 156 MADISON AVE READING PA 19605 (610) 921-0777

GOTTSCHALL FASHION PRODUCTION 1062 N 6TH ST READING PA 19601 (610) 373-2130

MARY LEISTER CHARM SCHOOL 539 CT ST READING PA 19601 (610) 373-6150

R-ACT PRODUCTIONS COMMUNITY 426 ADAMS ST ROCHESTER PA 15074 (412) 775-6844

BROADWAY THEATRE 108 N WASHINGTON AVE # 1103 SCRANTON PA 18503 (717) 342-7784

ED CURRY THEATRICAL AGENCY 371 N SUMNER AVE SCRANTON PA 18504 (717) 344-1087

HIGHLITE MODELING & CASTING 415 N 8TH AVE SCRANTON PA 18503 (717) 346-3166

EXCEL MODELING AGENCY 315 S ALLEN ST # 108 STATE COLLEGE PA 16801 (814) 234-3346

MARY LOU'S MODEL MANAGEMENT 34 S MAIN ST WILKES BARRE PA 18705 (717) 829-2011

IMAGE MAKERS CO 1406 3RD AVE YORK PA 17403 (717) 848-3783

Rhode Island

MODEL MANAGEMENT INC 900 PARK AVE CRANSTON RI 02910 (401) 941-3020

NINE MODELS 2968 E MAIN RD PORTSMOUTH RI 02871 (401) 682-2220

DONAHUE MODELS 14 ROME AVE PROVIDENCE RI 02904 (401) 353-4940

EXPOSURE AGENCY & STUDIO 43 ARNOLD AVE PROVIDENCE RI 02905 (401) 941-6611

MODEL CLUB 355 S WATER ST PROVIDENCE RI 02903 (401) 273-7120

JOHN CASABLANCAS MODEL MGMT 1 LAMBERT LIND HWY WARWICK RI 02886 (401) 463-5866

RHODE ISLAND MODEL AGENCY INC 725 W SHORE RD WARWICK RI 02889 (401) 739-2151

SOUTH CAROLINA

SHOW PEOPLE TALENT AGENCY 215 E BAY ST CHARLESTON SC 29401 (803) 727-0335

BUFFETTE MODELS WORKSHOP 1900 MARSHALL ST COLUMBIA SC 29203 (803) 779-7732

COLLINS MODELS-STUDIO & AGENCY 1441 GREENHILL RD COLUMBIA SC 29206 (803) 782-5223

CORE BOOKING AGENCY 238 S MARION ST COLUMBIA SC 29205 (803) 256-9300

HARVEST TALENT 2800 BUSH RIVER RD COLUMBIA SC 29210 (803) 798-4840

JUNIOR MISS SOUTH CAROLINA 6801 ST ANDREWS RD COLUMBIA SC 29212 (803) 732-4611

*MILLIE LEWIS OF COLUMBIA INC 3612 LANDMARK DR COLUMBIA SC 29204 (803) 782-7338

REVELATIONS MODELING TALENT 6701 TWO NOTCH RD COLUMBIA SC 29223 (803) 736-4586

SOUTH CAROLINA CASTING 5516 LAKESHORE DR COLUMBIA SC 29206 (803) 738-9003

SOUTHEASTERN TALENT BANK 3008 MILLWOOD AVE COLUMBIA SC 29205 (803) 765-1001

WILLIAM PETTIT TALENT AGENCY 4716 BRENTHAVEN RD COLUMBIA SC 29206 (803) 787-3113

MILLIE LEWIS SALON 1228 S PLEASANTBURG DR GREENVILLE SC 29605 (864) 299-1301

*MILLIE LEWIS MODELING 49 S FOREST BEACH DR # 110 HILTON HEAD ISLE SC 29928 (803) 785-6101

REFLECTIONS BY GA CROLLEY 7715 ST ANDREWS RD IRMO SC 29063 (803) 732-0634

SAME AGENCY 4550 LADSON RD LADSON SC 29456 (803) 871-0952

AFTERDECK 9719 HWY 17 N MYRTLE BEACH SC 29572 (803) 449-1550

BEVERLY HILLS TALENT MGMT 9719 HWY 17 N MYRTLE BEACH SC 29572 (803) 449-3655

MODEL SHOP 312 N KINGS HWY MYRTLE BEACH SC 29577 (803) 448-9860

SHOWPEOPLE TALENT AGENCY 1107 N 48TH AVE # 310F MYRTLE BEACH SC 29577 (803) 449-3895

NOUVEAU PRODUCTIONS 701 EDGEFIELD RD NORTH AUGUSTA SC 29841 (803) 441-0106

SHOWCASE MODELS 1200 33RD AVE S NORTH MYRTLE BCH SC 29582 (803) 272-8009

BETTY LANE SCHOOL OF CHARM 250 DOYLE ST SE ORANGEBURG SC 29115 (803) 534-9672

L H FIELDS GROUP 401 E KENNEDY ST SPARTANBURG SC 29302 (864) 591-0241

RUSSELL ADAIR FASHION STUDIO 1112 MEETING ST WEST COLUMBIA SC 29169 (803) 794-7233

SOUTH DAKOTA

BERNICE JOHNSON INTL SCHOOL 1320 S MINNESOTA AVE SIOUX FALLS SD 57105 (605) 338-3918

HAUTE MODELS MODELING SCHOOL 1002 W 6TH ST SIOUX FALLS SD 57104 (605) 334-6110

PROFESSIONAL IMAGE BY ROSEMARY 2815 E 26TH ST SIOUX FALLS SD 57103 (605) 334-0619

TENNESSEE

FINESSE MODELING SCHL & TALENT 115 BLACKLEY RD BRISTOL TN 37620 (423) 968-3406

AMBIANCE MODELING CTR 5959 SHALLOWFORD RD # 405 CHATTANOOGA TN 37421 (423) 499-1994

EVERGREEN AGENCY 100 CHEROKEE BLVD CHATTANOOGA TN 37405 (423) 266-1190

ACTION MODELING & TALENT AGNCY 500 PICKENS LN COLUMBIA TN 38401 (615) 381-8033

NORTH AMERICA MODELING 101 LYNNBROOK CT COLUMBIA TN 38401 (615) 381-5740

BARBIZON SCHOOL OF MODELING 6685 POPLAR AVE # 04 GERMANTOWN TN 38138 (901) 755-6800

TALENT AGENCY INC 1005 LAVERGNE CIR HENDERSONVILLE TN 37075 (615) 822-1143

MODEL WORLD 19 NORTHSTAR RD JACKSON TN 38305 (901) 661-9551

18 KARAT TALENT & MODELING 6409 DEANE HILL DR KNOXVILLE TN 37919 (423) 558-0004

MODEL SEARCH 8905 KINGSTON PIKE KNOXVILLE TN 37923 (423) 453-1444

PREMIER MODELS & TALENT 5201 KINGSTON PIKE KNOXVILLE TN 37919 (423) 694-7073

TALENT TREK 406 11TH ST KNOXVILLE TN 37916 (423) 977-8735

ADANTE'S MODELING 2364 KIMBALL AVE MEMPHIS TN 38114 (901) 744-0165

CARVEL MODEL & TALENT AGENCY 7075 POPLAR AVE MEMPHIS TN 38138 (901) 754-4747

COLORS TALENT AGENCY 269 S FRONT ST MEMPHIS TN 38103 (901) 523-9900

*DONNA GROFF AGENCY INC PO BOX 382517 MEMPHIS TN 38183 (901) 854-5561

MODEL & TALENT MANAGEMENT 6263 POPLAR AVE MEMPHIS TN 38119 (901) 685-0079

ROBBINS MODELS & TALENT 1213 PARK PLACE MALL # 246 MEMPHIS TN 38119 (901) 753-8360

SACTO BOOKING AGENT 3355 POPLAR AVE MEMPHIS TN 38111 (901) 458-2909

ACT INC 3840 DICKERSON RD NASHVILLE TN 37207 (615) 865-8330

ADVANTAGE MODELS & TALENT 4825 TROUSDALE DR # 230 NASHVILLE TN 37220 (615) 833-3005

AGENCY 20 MUSIC SQ W NASHVILLE TN 37203 (615) 371-0233

AMAX 4121 HILLSBORO RD NASHVILLE TN 37215 (615) 292-0246

AMERICAN TALENT AGENCY 1300 DIVISION ST NASHVILLE TN 37203 (615) 259-9333

ARTIST DIRECTION AGENCY 2011 RICHARD JONES RD NASHVILLE TN 37215 (615) 383-9136

BARBIZON SCHOOL OF MODELING 2000 GLEN ECHO RD # 207 NASHVILLE TN 37215 (615) 298-4402

CENTURY II PROMOTIONS 523 HEATHER PL NASHVILLE TN 37204 (615) 385-5700

FLAIR MODELS 672 LAKE TERRACE DR NASHVILLE TN 37217 (615) 361-3737

FROM THE HEART TALENT 224 THOMPSON LN NASHVILLE TN 37211 (615) 831-2042

GO FISH BOOKING 609 MERRITT AVE NASHVILLE TN 37203 (615) 385-7999

HARPER AGENCY 4004 HILLSBORO RD NASHVILLE TN 37215 (615) 383-1455

J HARDY & ASSOC 50 MUSIC SQ W NASHVILLE TN 37203 (615) 329-2881

JO-SUSAN 2817 W END AVE NASHVILLE TN 37203 (615) 327-8726

KANINE KONTROL 3531 CENTRAL AVE NASHVILLE TN 37205 (615) 385-4592

KEY TALENT INC 1808 W END AVE NASHVILLE TN 37203 (615) 242-2461

KUP CASTING 705 18TH AVE S NASHVILLE TN 37203 (615) 327-0181

MADISON AGENCY 240 OLD HICKORY BLVD NASHVILLE TN 37221 (615) 865-6543

MC HUGH MANAGEMENT PO BOX 41647 NASHVILLE TN 37204 (615) 889-1474

MISS TENNESSEE USA DIRECTOR PO BOX 140692 NASHVILLE TN 37214 (615) 889-2443

MRS TENNESSEE USI PAGENT 3904 WALLACE LN NASHVILLE TN 37215 (615) 661-0804

OPRY LINK MODELING & TALENT 50 MUSIC SQ W NASHVILLE TN 37203 (615) 320-9501

TALENT CONNECTION CASTING 411 COVENTRY DR NASHVILLE TN 37211 (615) 831-0039

TML TALENT AGENCY-TALENT 705 18TH AVE S NASHVILLE TN 37203 (615) 321-5596

U S TALENT AGENCY 60 MUSIC SQ W NASHVILLE TN 37203 (615) 327-2255

MODEL SEARCH 1902 WINFIELD DUNN PKY SEVIERVILLE TN 37876 (423) 453-1489

TEXAS

DIANE'S SCHOOL OF MODELING 1410 S WASHINGTON ST AMARILLO TX 79102 (806) 376-8936

MODELS WEST 2201 S WESTERN ST # 121 AMARILLO TX 79109 (806) 352-1943

SELECT MODELING & TALENT 3405 S WESTERN ST AMARILLO TX 79109 (806) 352-1173

ACCLAIM 4107 MED PKY # 210 AUSTIN TX 78756 (512) 323-5566

CIAO TALENTS 11303 SLIPPERY ELM TRL AUSTIN TX 78750 (512) 918-2426

CLASS 3603 SOUTHRIDGE DR AUSTIN TX 78704 (512) 450-1114

D B TALENT 3107 W SLAUGHTER LN AUSTIN TX 78748 (512) 892-7814

K HALL MODELS & TALENT 101 W 6TH ST AUSTIN TX 78701 (512) 476-7523

INFINITY MODELING & TALENT 4838 HOLLY RD # 206 CORPUS CHRISTI TX 78411 (512) 985-6191

REFLECTIONS INC TALENT 3817 S ALAMEDA ST CORPUS CHRISTI TX 78411 (512) 857-5414

PEGGY GREEN CAREER & MODELING 1813 MONTE VISTA ST DALHART TX 79022 (806) 249-8036

ANNE O'BRIANT AGENCY 3101 N FITZHUGH AVE # 301 DALLAS TX 75204 (214) 871-7568

CAMPBELL AGENCY 3906 LEMMON AVE DALLAS TX 75219 (214) 522-8991

CLIPSE MODEL & TALENT MGMT 3624 OAKLAWN AVE, STE 300 DALLAS TX 75219 (214) 520-6150

DALLAS MODEL GROUP 12700 HILLCREST RD DALLAS TX 75230 (972) 980-7647

ELAN MODEL & TALENT MANAGEMENT 4215 MCEWEN RD DALLAS TX 75244 (972) 239-2398

ELECTRIC ARTISTS 5722 GOODWIN AVE DALLAS TX 75206 (214) 824-3825

GCC DALLAS TALENT & MODEL 3136 ROUTH ST DALLAS TX 75201 (214) 220-0217

HENNIE & CO 2351 W HWY DALLAS TX 75220 (214) 350-5898

JOHN ROBERT POWERS MODELING 13601 PRESTON RD # 4 DALLAS TX 75240 (972) 239-9551

JOY WYSE AGENCY 406 NEWELL AVE DALLAS TX 75223 (214) 319-9973

*KIM DAWSON AGENCY, INC. 2300 STEMMONS FREEWAY #1643 DALLAS TX 75207 (214) 638-2414

MARY COLLINS AGENCY 5956 SHERRY LN # 917 DALLAS TX 75225 (214) 360-0900

MIRAGE MODELING 2210 IRVING BLVD DALLAS TX 75207 (214) 741-0702

*PAGE PARKES MODELS REP 3303 LEE PKY DALLAS TX 75219 (214) 526-4434

PEGGY TAYLOR TALENT INC 1825 MARKET CTR DALLAS TX 75207 (214) 651-7884

TALENT SCOUT 8350 N CENTRAL EXPY DALLAS TX 75206 (214) 691-8680

TOMAS AGENCY 240 TURNPIKE AVE DALLAS TX 75208 (214) 943-5181

TR TALENT RESOURCES 9550 SKILLMAN ST DALLAS TX 75243 (214) 343-3003

DENTON COMMUNITY THEATRE 214 W HICKORY ST DENTON TX 76201 (817) 382-7014

FACES DEMO AGENCY 1701 OAKS RD EDINBURG TX 78539 (210) 380-3455

FRAN SIMON MODEL & TALENT AGCY 9619 ACER AVE EL PASO TX 79925 (915) 594-8772

JOHN CASABLANCA'S MODELING 8901 MCFALL DR EL PASO TX 79925 (915) 598-9899

TALENT HOUSE 808 N EUCALYPTUS ST EL PASO TX 79903 (915) 533-1945

ACTOR'S PREPARATORY STUDIO 1020 W 7TH ST FORT WORTH TX 76102 (817) 335-2281

ACTORS PREPARATORY STUDIO 901 LAKE ST # 40 FORT WORTH TX 76102 (817) 334-0800

BARBIZON MODELS 4950 OVERTON RIDGE BLVD FORT WORTH TX 76132 (817) 294-0554

MODELS GROUP AGENCY 6322 CAMP BOWIE BLVD FORT WORTH TX 76116 (817) 738-2029

DANIEL-HORNE AGENCY 1576 NO HWY GARLAND TX 75041 (972) 613-7827

TALENT EXPRESS 602 COLLEGE ST GRAND PRAIRIE TX 75050 (972) 642-3201

GABRIELLE'S 543 W VETERANS MEMORIAL BLVD HARKER HEIGHTS TX 76548 (817) 699-8075

ACTORS ETC INC 2620 FOUNTAIN VIEW DR # 210 HOUSTON TX 77057 (713) 785-4495

BARBIZON 621 WELLESLEY DR HOUSTON TX 77024 (713) 850-9111

BARBIZON SCHOOL OF MODELING 5433 WESTHEIMER RD # 300 HOUSTON TX 77056 (713) 850-9111

FIRST MODELS & TALENT AGENCY 5433 WESTHEIMER RD # 305 HOUSTON TX 77056 (713) 850-9611

INTER-MEDIA MODEL & TALENT 5353 W ALABAMA ST # 222 HOUSTON TX 77056 (713) 622-8282

MAD HATTER MODEL & TALENT   2620 FOUNTAIN VIEW DR # 212 HOUSTON TX 77057 (713) 266-5800

MISS TEXAS USA PAGEANT 820 GESSNER RD HOUSTON TX 77024 (713) 461-4600

NEAL HAMIL AGENCY 7887 SAN FELIPE ST HOUSTON TX 77063 (713) 789-1335

PAGE PARKES SCHOOL OF MODELING 5353 W. ALABAMA, #220 HOUSTON TX 77056 (713) 622-7171

UNIVERSAL TALENT 5601 ARLINGTON ST HOUSTON TX 77076 (713) 691-2222

YOUNG ARTISTS 12330 BRAEWICK DR HOUSTON TX 77035 (713) 847-8900

IVETT STONE AGENCY INC 6309 N O CONNOR BLVD IRVING TX 75039 (972) 506-9962

JON' TAY MODELING & THEATRICAL 3353 GILMER RD LONGVIEW TX 75604 (903) 297-9189

SHERITA LYNNE MODELING AGENCY 320 RUTHLYNN DR LONGVIEW TX 75605 (903) 758-1259

ROBERT SPENCE SCHOOL 4418 74TH ST # 53 LUBBOCK TX 79424 (806) 797-8134

AVANT MODELS & CASTING 85 NE LOOP 410 # 218A SAN ANTONIO TX 78216 (210) 308-8411

CONDRA/ARTISTA MODELING   13300 OLD BLANCO RD # 201 SAN ANTONIO TX 78216 (210) 492-9947

SINCLAIR TALENT INTL 4115 MED DR # 401 SAN ANTONIO TX 78229 (210) 614-2281

UTAH

FINISHING TOUCH 3725 WASHINGTON BLVD OGDEN UT 84403 (801) 394-3771

ALMA MATER 68 S MAIN ST # 612 SALT LAKE CITY UT 84101 (801) 575-7075

BARBIZON SCHOOL OF MODELING 1363 S STATE ST # 232 SALT LAKE CITY UT 84115 (801) 487-7591

EASTMAN AGENCY 560 W 200 S SALT LAKE CITY UT 84101 (801) 364-8434

ELITE MEDIA MODEL & TALENT INC 749 S STATE ST SALT LAKE CITY UT 84111 (801) 539-1740

HAILE TALENT AGENCY INC 366 S 500 E SALT LAKE CITY UT 84102 (801) 532-6961

KLC TALENT INC 772 W TEMPLE SALT LAKE CITY UT 84104 (801) 364-7447

LINDSAY WALKER 2227 E BRIDGEWATER SALT LAKE CITY UT 84121 (801) 942-2660

MC CARTY SALONS 1326 FOOTHILL DR SALT LAKE CITY UT 84108 (801) 581-9911

PREMIERE MODELS 817 E 2100 S SALT LAKE CITY UT 84106 (801) 466-8539

ROCKET AGENCY 1019 E 2700 S SALT LAKE CITY UT 84106 (801) 485-2505

STYLE INC 560 W 200 S SALT LAKE CITY UT 84101 (801) 539-7703

SUSIE'S MODELING & DANCE STD 635 E 100 # 3 SALT LAKE CITY UT 84102 (801) 363-4956

UTAH TALENT FIND 3948 PINETREE DR SALT LAKE CITY UT 84124 (801) 944-4431

EXECUTIVE MODEL SHOP 9480 UNION SQ # 203 SANDY UT 84070 (801) 572-5300

SUSIE KUBY-MILLER'S MODELING 273 E 2100 S SOUTH SALT LAKE UT 84115 (801) 487-4238

VIRGINIA

ENCORE MODEL & TALENT AGENCY 826 RIVERGATE PL ALEXANDRIA VA 22314 (703) 548-0900

MODEL & TALENT MANAGEMENT 249 S VAN DORN ST ALEXANDRIA VA 22304 (703) 823-5203

TEAM GUSTAFSON 946 FERRYMAN QUAY CHESAPEAKE VA 23323 (757) 485-1201

BARONE & CO 5599 SEMINARY RD FALLS CHURCH VA 22041 (703) 768-2231

FOX ENTERPRISES INC 7700 LEESBURG PIKE # 100 FALLS CHURCH VA 22043 (703) 506-0335

ERICKSON AGENCY 1491 CHAIN BRIDGE RD # 200 MC LEAN VA 22101 (703) 356-0040

TALENT MANAGEMENT 1481 CHAIN BRIDGE RD MC LEAN VA 22101 (703) 356-8357

MARILYN'S-THE PROFESSIONAL 2721 CHARTSTONE DR MIDLOTHIAN VA 23113 (804) 379-1946

WRIGHT MODELING AGENCY 12638 JEFFERSON AVE # 16 NEWPORT NEWS VA 23602 (757) 886-5884

NEW YORK MODELING AGENCY 1225 BOISSEVAIN AVE NORFOLK VA 23507 (757) 626-3880

TALENT CONNECTION INC 809 BRANDON AVE # 300 NORFOLK VA 23517 (757) 624-1975

FOXX FIRE FASHION SHOWS PO BOX 26572 RICHMOND VA 23261 (804) 329-5190

MODEL SHOPPE 1203 W MAIN ST RICHMOND VA 23220 (804) 278-8743

MODELOGIC 2501 E BROAD ST RICHMOND VA 23223 (804) 644-1000

STUDIOS LTD MODEL-TALENT NET 118 CAMPBELL AVE SE ROANOKE VA 24011 (540) 345-6300

WINNING IMAGE GROUP 556 GARRISONVILLE RD STAFFORD VA 22554 (540) 720-4643

NEW FACES MODELS 8230 LEESBURG PIKE # 520 VIENNA VA 22182 (703) 821-0786

CHARM ASSOCIATES INC 144 BUSINESS PARK DR # 100 VIRGINIA BEACH VA 23462 (757) 490-8340

EVIE MANSFIELD MODELING 505 S INDEPENDENCE BLVD # 205 VIRGINIA BCH VA 23452 (757) 490-5990

STEINHART-NORTON TALENT MGMT 312 ARCTIC CRES VIRGINIA BEACH VA 23451 (757) 422-8535

WINNING MODELS 3824 VIRGINIA BEACH BLVD VIRGINIA BEACH VA 23452 (757) 631-0307

XTRA TALENT 1110 ATLANTIC AVE VIRGINIA BEACH VA 23451 (757) 425-7220

BARBIZON SCHOOL OF MODELING 609 CEDAR CREEK GRADE WINCHESTER VA 22601 (540) 662-2222

VERMONT

DEBRA LEWIN PRODUCTIONS & TLNT 269 PEARL ST BURLINGTON VT 05401 (802) 865-2234

WASHINGTON

ABC KIDS PERFORMING ARTS CTR 924 BELLEVUE WAY NE BELLEVUE WA 98004 (206) 646-5440

E L VOGUE INT'L MODELS INC 400 NE 108TH AVE # 604 BELLEVUE WA 98004 (206) 688-8183

JOHN CASABLANCAS MODEL & TLNT 155 NE 108TH AVE # 600 BELLEVUE WA 98004 (206) 646-3585

JTM KIDS & TEENS 411 108TH AVE NE BELLEVUE WA 98004 (206) 454-3677

KID BIZ TALENT AGENCY 411 NE 108TH AVE # 2050 BELLEVUE WA 98004 (206) 455-8800

DOUGLASS MODELS & MEDIA 3881 MAGRATH RD BELLINGHAM WA 98226 (360) 647-0716

MODELS NORTHWEST INTL 1227 PUGET ST BELLINGHAM WA 98226 (360) 647-3326

TEAM MODELS 3431 96TH AVE NE CLYDE HILL WA 98004 (206) 455-2969

SUNNY'S MODEL DEV AGENCY 23830 HWY 99 EDMONDS WA 98026 (206) 670-2171

TCM MODELS 4415 W CLEARWATER AVE KENNEWICK WA 99336 (509) 783-5868

ALLEINAD MODELING AGENCY 147 ROGERS ST NW OLYMPIA WA 98502 (360) 705-2573

ACTORS & WALKER 600 1ST AVE SEATTLE WA 98104 (206) 682-4368

ACTORS GROUP 114 S ALASKAN WAY # 104 SEATTLE WA 98104 (206) 624-9465

BABY MODEL OF AMERICA 1463 E REPUBLICAN ST # 300 SEATTLE WA 98112 (206) 322-2215

BARBIZON SCHOOL OF MODELING 1501 4TH AVE # 305 SEATTLE WA 98101 (206) 223-1500

CAROL JAMES TALENT AGENCY 117 S MAIN ST SEATTLE WA 98104 (206) 447-9191

DRAMATIC ARTISTS/DRAMATIC KIDS 1000 LENORA ST # 511 SEATTLE WA 98121 (206) 442-9190

E THOMAS BLISS & ASSOC 219 1ST AVE S SEATTLE WA 98104 (206) 340-1875

EDGE MODEL MANAGEMENT 911 E PIKE ST SEATTLE WA 98122 (206) 860-8874

EILEEN SEALS INTL 600 STEWART ST SEATTLE WA 98101 (206) 448-2040

FUTURE STARS TOTS N TEENS MDL 17900 SOUTHCENTER PKY # 200 SEATTLE WA 98188 (206) 575-7922

HEFFNER TALENT AGENCY 1601 5TH AVE # 2301 SEATTLE WA 98101 (206) 622-2211

KIDS TEAM 911 E PIKE ST SEATTLE WA 98122 (206) 860-8688

KIM BROOKE GROUP 2044 EASTLAKE AVE E SEATTLE WA 98102 (206) 329-1111

LOLA HALLOWELL TALENT AGENCY 1700 N WESTLAKE AVE # 702 SEATTLE WA 98109 (206) 281-4646

MATURE TALENT ENTERPRISES 620 W 5TH AVE # 109 SEATTLE WA 98119 (206) 283-3367

RICHARD'S AGENCY INTL USA 720 OLIVE WAY SEATTLE WA 98101 (206) 467-1989

SEATTLE MODELS GUILD 1809 7TH AVE SEATTLE WA 98101 (206) 622-1406

TALENT AGENCY 89 YESLER WAY SEATTLE WA 98104 (206) 624-7245

TCM INC 2200 6TH AVE # 100 SEATTLE WA 98121 (206) 728-4826

THOMPSON MEDIA TALENT 11522 24TH AVE NE SEATTLE WA 98125 (206) 363-5555

TOPO SWOPE TALENT AGENCY 1932 1ST AVE SEATTLE WA 98101 (206) 443-2021

TRAINING CENTER FOR MODELS 2200 6TH AVE # 100 SEATTLE WA 98121 (206) 728-1810

CHELSEA CHARM & MDLNG STUDIO 221 N WALL ST SPOKANE WA 99201 (509) 624-5971

P J & CO MODELS & FINISHING 9612 E SPRAGUE AVE SPOKANE WA 99206 (509) 922-8102

P J & CO SCHOOL OF FASHION 9612 E SPRAGUE AVE SPOKANE WA 99206 (509) 922-9102

ABC KIDS 10828 GRAVELLY LAKE DR SW TACOMA WA 98499 (206) 581-2680

ANDERSEN MODELS INTL 3030 68TH AVE W TACOMA WA 98466 (206) 564-5830

WISCONSIN

A & M TALENT CASTING 3110 W SPENCER ST APPLETON WI 54914 (414) 731-6088

MODEL MANAGEMENT INC 101 W EDISON AVE APPLETON WI 54915 (414) 733-1212

MODEL CONNECTION 3629 MORMON COULEE RD LA CROSSE WI 54601 (608) 788-9300

BOOM MANAGEMENT PO BOX 9632 MADISON WI 53725 (608) 257-2007

GERED MODELS INTL LTD 2702 MONROE ST MADISON WI 53711 (608) 238-6372

K C TALENT 301 S BEDFORD ST MADISON WI 53703 (608) 257-2577

LORI LINS LTD 700 RAY O VAC DR MADISON WI 53711 (608) 274-8100

MODEL EXCHANGE LTD 3769 E WASHINGTON AVE MADISON WI 53704 (608) 241-1700

*ARLENE WILSON MANAGEMENT 809 S 60TH ST # 201 MILWAUKEE WI 53214 (414) 778-3838

BULLOCK & ASSOC LTD PO BOX 92516 MILWAUKEE WI 53202 (414) 272-2345

CREATIVE ASSOCIATES 5401 W PRESIDIO LN MILWAUKEE WI 53223 (414) 353-1018

JENNIFER'S TALENT UNLIMITED 740 N PLANKINTON AVE MILWAUKEE WI 53203 (414) 277-9440

JOHN ROBERT POWERS MODELING 700 N WATER ST MILWAUKEE WI 53202 (414) 273-4468

LORI LINS LTD 7611 W HOLMES AVE MILWAUKEE WI 53220 (414) 282-3500

MIDWEST TALENT PRODUCTIONS 1726 N 1ST ST MILWAUKEE WI 53212 (414) 374-3744

MISS BLACK WISCONSIN PAGEANT 927 E OGDEN AVE MILWAUKEE WI 53202 (414) 273-1115

POWERS MODEL MANAGEMENT 700 N WATER ST MILWAUKEE WI 53202 (414) 273-4470

Order Form

Yes, I want to invest $19.95 in my future! Send _____ copies of Modeling: Totally Exposed. Please add $3.00 postage and handling per book. (Florida residents add $1.40 sales tax.)

Name _____

Company _____

Address _____

City/State/Zip _____

❏ Check or money order enclosed. Charge my ❏ Visa ❏ Mastercard

Account# and Expiration Date _____

Signature _____

Please make your checks payable to:
Marsha Doll Models
P.O. Box 15814
Tallahassee, FL 32317-5814
(850) 656–7835
Quantity Discounts Available

NOTES

NOTES